Common Surgeries Made Easy

Efstathios Karamanos
Editor

Common Surgeries Made Easy

A Quick Guide for Residents and Medical Students

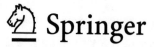 Springer

Editor
Efstathios Karamanos, MD
Plastic and Reconstructive Surgery
UT Health San Antonio
San Antonio, TX
USA

Assistant Editors

Arielle Hodari Gupta, MD
Associate program director
General Surgery
Henry Ford Hospital
Detroit, MI
USA

Noah Saad, MD
Division of Plastic and
Reconstructive Surgery
UT Health San Antonio
San Antonio, TX
USA

ISBN 978-3-030-41349-1 ISBN 978-3-030-41350-7 (eBook)
https://doi.org/10.1007/978-3-030-41350-7

This Springer imprint is published by the registered company Springer Nature Switzerland AG
The registered company address is: Gewerbestrasse 11, 6330 Cham, Switzerland

To my father, Konstantinos, and my mother, Angeliki, for their unmeasured, endless, and selfless support.
To all the unsung heroes around the world fighting with multiple sclerosis.
To the infinite white and blue of the Grecian land. And to all those who like Odysseus, are on their personal quest to find their own Ithaca.

Special thanks to
Bao-Quynh Julian, MD,
from the Division of Plastic and Reconstructive Surgery, UT Health San Antonio, for the illustrations throughout the book.

Arielle Hodari Gupta, MD,
Associate program director, General Surgery Henry Ford Hospital/Wayne State University, Detroit, MI

Noah Saad, MD,
Plastic and Reconstructive Surgery, UT Health San Antonio, San Antonio, TX

Preface

I vividly remember my first day as an intern in general surgery. It was a gloomy morning, and I was up since 3 a.m., excited to finally be a doctor. My chief resident looked at me and told me: "You go do the inguinal hernia today." My excitement was swiftly traded with pure terror: How can I be competent when I have no idea what I am supposed to be doing? I spent the next 2 hours researching every possible source I could find but was disappointed to find that there are no clear and precise resources to quickly and efficiently go through the steps of such a common operation. That day was the birth of the idea of the book you have in your hands today.

The present book tries to fulfill a need of medical students during their surgical rotations, of interns looking to understand common surgical procedures, and of chief residents reviewing steps for the most commonly asked operations during board certification. The book is written in a simple fashion, with bullet-point steps to be easy and quick for the reader. It also includes hints about the positioning of the patient and potential pitfalls for every surgery.

On behalf of all the authors, I hope that this book will become an invaluable companion, one that will be inside your white coat pocket, worn from use, and always your ally during the stressful days of surgical rotations and residency.

San Antonio, TX, USA   Efstathios Karamanos

Contents

Contributors

Imran Ahmad, MD Department of General Surgery, Henry Ford Hospital/Wayne State University, Detroit, MI, USA

Heath J. Antoine, MD Robert Wood Johnson University Hospital, New Brunswick, NJ, USA

Justin Chamberlain, MD ProMedica Physicians General Surgery, Monroe, MI, USA

Konstantinos Chouliaras, MD Department of Surgery, Wake Forest University, Winston-Salem, NC, USA

Megan A. Coughlin, MD Division of Pediatric Surgery, UT Health Science Center in Houston, Houston, TX, USA

Sophie Dream, MD Division of Surgical Oncology, University of Alabama, Birmingham, AL, USA

Marianne Franco, MD, FACS Henry Ford West Bloomfield Hospital, West Bloomfield, MI, USA

Claire Gerall, MD Department of Surgery, UT Health San Antonio, San Antonio, TX, USA

Arielle Hodari Gupta, MD Department of Surgery, Henry Ford Hospital/Wayne State University, Detroit, MI, USA

Tommy Ivanics, MD Department of General Surgery, Henry Ford Hospital/Wayne State University, Detroit, MI, USA

Efstathios Karamanos, MD Plastic and Reconstructive Surgery, UT Health San Antonio, San Antonio, TX, USA

Yasaman Kavousi, MD Department of General Surgery, Henry Ford Hospital/Wayne State University, Detroit, MI, USA

Mio Kitano, MD Division of Surgical Oncology and Endocrine Surgery, UT Health San Antonio, San Antonio, TX, USA

Shravan Leonard-Murali, MD Department of Surgery, Henry Ford Hospital/Wayne State University, Detroit, MI, USA

Sanjay Mohanty, MD Division of Colon and Rectal Surgery, Barnes-Jewish Hospital, St. Louis, MO, USA

Semeret T. Munie, MD Division of Bariatric and Minimally Invasive Surgery, Medical College of Wisconsin, Milwaukee, WI, USA

Hassan Nasser, MD Department of General Surgery, Henry Ford Hospital/Wayne State University, Detroit, MI, USA

Puraj Patel, DO Henry Ford West Bloomfield Hospital, West Bloomfield, MI, USA

Michael Rizzari, MD Division of Transplant and Hepatobiliary Surgery, Henry Ford Hospital/Wayne State University, Detroit, MI, USA

Nicholas Robbins, DO Department of Surgery, UT Health San Antonio, San Antonio, TX, USA

Kelly Rosso, MD Department of Surgical Oncology, Banner MD Anderson Cancer Center, Gilbert, AZ, USA

Amita Shah, MD Division of Plastic and Reconstructive Surgery, UT Health San Antonio, San Antonio, TX, USA

Rupen Shah Division of Surgical Oncology, Department of Surgery, Henry Ford Hospital/Wayne State University, Detroit, MI, USA

Ryan Shelden, DO Division of Acute Care Surgery and Critical Care, Henry Ford Hospital/Wayne State University, Detroit, MI, USA

Michael Sippel, MD Department of Surgery, UT Health San Antonio, San Antonio, TX, USA

Mallory Wampler, MD Department of Surgery, UT Health San Antonio, San Antonio, TX, USA

Adam Wandell, DDS Department of Oral and Maxillofacial Surgery, UT Health San Antonio, San Antonio, TX, USA

Shawn Webb, MD Division of Colon and Rectal Surgery, Henry Ford Hospital/Wayne State University, Detroit, MI, USA

Jaclyn Yracheta, MD Department of Surgery, UT Health San Antonio, San Antonio, TX, USA

Part I
Esophagus

Chapter 1
Laparoscopic Nissen Fundoplication

Yasaman Kavousi

Overview

- Dissection through gastrohepatic ligament
- Identify right crus, and dissect posteriorly
- Takedown short gastrics working cranially towards left crus
- Complete circumferential mobilization of esophagus
- Closure of hiatus if needed
- Fundus passed posteriorly and wrap created and sewn in place with 3 stitches

Clinical Pearls

- Replaced left hepatic artery courses through gastrohepatic ligament
- Left vagus nerve courses anterior, right vagus nerve courses posterior
- If not using bougie, can use gastroscope to assess tightness of wrap

Y. Kavousi (✉)
Department of General Surgery,
Henry Ford Hospital/Wayne State University, Detroit, MI, USA
e-mail: ykavousi@hfhs.org

© Springer Nature Switzerland AG 2020
E. Karamanos (ed.), *Common Surgeries Made Easy*,
https://doi.org/10.1007/978-3-030-41350-7_1

- Patient may have dysphagia immediately postoperatively secondary to swelling, inflammation but will resolve with time

Patient Preparation

Supine with both arms tucked by his/her side.

After induction of general anesthesia, an orogastric tube and an optional urinary catheter are placed.

Anesthesia

General anesthesia.

Operative Steps

1. Pneumoperitoneum is established using a Veress needle technique via a supra-umbilical incision to the left of the midline (refer to chapter regarding abdominal entry).
2. A 10 mm laparoscope is then inserted and the peritoneal space is carefully inspected.
3. The remaining ports are placed sequentially under direct visualization, including a 5 mm self-retaining liver retractor, utilizing a five-port technique.
4. The left lobe of the liver is elevated.
5. The patient is placed in steep reverse Trendelenburg position.
6. With the stomach retracted laterally, dissection commences by dividing the gastrohepatic ligament above the hepatic branch of the vagus (pars flaccida) using the Harmonic scalpel. Care is taken to avoid the left gastric artery, a possible replaced left hepatic artery, and vagal branches.
7. The right diaphragmatic crus is identified and the overlying peritoneal attachments are divided.

8. The right crus is dissected from its confluence to the median arcuate ligament, where it joins the left crus posterior to the esophagus.
9. The phrenoesophageal membrane is carefully divided anteriorly, perpendicular to the esophagus.
10. The anterior vagus nerve is generally affixed to the esophagus, and the posterior vagus nerve is not visible at this time.
11. Next, the stomach is grasped at the level of the inferior pole of the spleen. The greater omentum is also grasped and retracted laterally.
12. Using the Harmonic scalpel, the short gastric vessels along the greater curvature are divided to the level of the left diaphragmatic crus.
13. The esophagus is freed from the left crus and mobilized circumferentially at the hiatus. Great care is taken to avoid injury to the esophagus, stomach and vagus nerve.
14. The gastroesophageal junction is identified by recognizing the confluence of the longitudinal muscles of the esophagus merging with the sling muscles of the stomach.
15. In the majority of patients, adequate intra-abdominal esophagus is present and an esophageal lengthening procedure is not needed.
16. A 56 French bougie is passed by Anesthesia through the esophagus along the lesser curvature of the stomach.
17. The esophagus is retracted with the help of a penrose drain and the hiatal confluence is closed by bringing the left and right crux together, posterior to the esophagus. The crura are sewn to each other moving from the patient's left side to the right side with interrupted 0 Ethibond suture using the Endostitch device.
18. The fundus of the stomach is then passed behind the esophagus.
19. A shoeshine maneuver is performed to ensure correct alignment, tension, and placement of the wrap.
20. With the bougie in place, a 2 cm 360 degree wrap is created and secured with 3 interrupted 0 Ethibond sutures using the Endostitch device.

21. Sutures are passed from the fundus on the left side of the wrap to the esophagus and then to the fundus on the right side of the wrap. The most distal sutures may incorporate only the fundus to fundus. An additional two sutures may be placed from the fundus on the right side posteriorly to the right crus to further anchor the wrap (Fig. 1.1).
22. The bougie is then removed and the repair is inspected visually to ensure that the wrap is configured correctly.
23. All ports are removed and pneumoperitoneum is evacuated and the skin incisions closed.

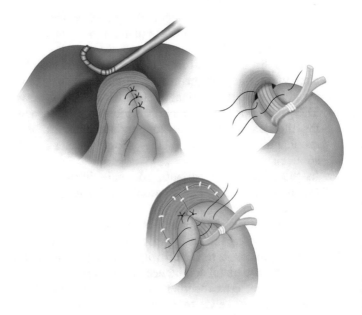

FIGURE 1.1 Three interrupted 0 Ethibond sutures are placed at the fundus of the stomach around a 56 French Bougie

Chapter 2
Minimally Invasive Heller Myotomy

Yasaman Kavousi

Overview

- Dissection through gastrohepatic ligament
- Identify right crus, and dissect posteriorly
- Complete circumferential mobilization of esophagus
- Identify anterior vagus nerve and protect
- Myotomy should extend through muscle to see mucosa

  - 8 cm onto esophagus, and at least 2 cm onto stomach cardia

Clinical Pearls

- Replaced left hepatic artery courses through gastrohepatic ligament
- Left vagus nerve courses anterior, right vagus nerve courses posterior
- If patients need anti-reflux surgery, attending preference for anterior or posterior wrap

Y. Kavousi (✉)
Department of General Surgery,
Henry Ford Hospital/Wayne State University, Detroit, MI, USA
e-mail: ykavousi@hfhs.org

© Springer Nature Switzerland AG 2020   7
E. Karamanos (ed.), *Common Surgeries Made Easy*,
https://doi.org/10.1007/978-3-030-41350-7_2

- Anterior wrap benefit: protects the mucosa, and will cover any possible missed mucosal injuries
- Posterior wrap benefits: stents the esophagus open to avoid future dysphagia

Patient Preparation

Supine with both arms tucked by his/her side.

After induction of general anesthesia, an optional urinary catheter is placed.

Anesthesia

General anesthesia.

Operative Steps

1. The skin of the lower chest and abdomen is prepped and draped in the usual sterile fashion.
2. The peritoneal cavity is accessed using a Veress needle via a supra-umbilical incision and pneumoperitoneum is established.
3. A 10 mm laparoscope is then inserted, and the intra-peritoneal cavity is evaluated.
4. The laparoscopic ports include either a 5 mm or 10 mm port placed 15 cm below the xiphoid and to the left of the midline. A 30-degree laparoscope is placed through this port and four additional ports are placed: two 5 mm ports below costal margin on each side and 15 cm away from the xiphoid, a 5 mm and 10 mm port on the right side and left side respectively and 10 cm away from the xiphoid and about 3–4 cm away from the midline.

5. The patient is placed in reverse Trendelenburg and a self-retaining liver retractor is placed through the right costal margin port (under the lateral segment of the left lobe of the liver to expose the hiatus). The robot is then docked if the surgery is being performed robotically, and the senior surgeon will scrub out to sit at the console.
6. Dissection begins by incising the gastrohepatic omentum to identify the right diaphragmatic crus.
7. The esophagus is then circumferentially dissected in the mediastinum by clearing the retroesophageal window and identifying the left diaphragmatic crus.
8. The gastroesophageal fat pad is then divided to expose the gastroesophageal junction. The vagus nerve is identified. Care is taken not to injure the nerve.
9. A 56 French bougie is then introduced into the esophagus.
10. The myotomy is then carried out using hook electrocautery. It is extended proximally a distance of 8 cm on the esophagus and distally a distance of 2 cm onto the cardia with care taken not to violate the mucosa (Fig. 2.1).
11. Approximately 50% of the esophageal circumference should be exposed.
12. The bougie is then withdrawn.
13. All ports are removed and pneumoperitoneum is evacuated. The fascia at the 10 mm port sites is closed and the skin is closed.
14. A sterile dressing is applied.

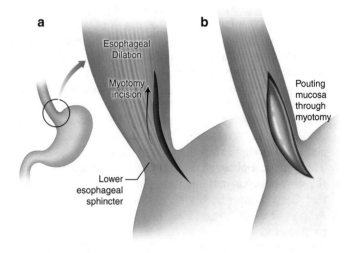

FIGURE 2.1 The Heller myotomy is performed using electrocautery 8 cm proximal to the esophagus and 2 cm distal to the stomach

Chapter 3
Laparoscopic Transabdominal Paraesophageal Hernia Repair

Semeret T. Munie

Overview

- Dissection through gastrohepatic ligament
- Identify right crus, and dissect posteriorly
- Takedown short gastrics working cranially towards left crus
- Complete circumferential mobilization of esophagus
- Hernia sac dissected out of mediastinum
- Hiatus primarily repaired with nonaborbable sutures
- Anti-reflux procedure is performed

Clinical Pearls

- Replaced left hepatic artery can run through gastrohepatic ligament
- Left vagus nerve courses anterior, right vagus nerve courses posterior

S. T. Munie (✉)
Division of Bariatric and Minimally Invasive Surgery, Medical College of Wisconsin, Milwaukee, WI, USA

© Springer Nature Switzerland AG 2020
E. Karamanos (ed.), *Common Surgeries Made Easy*, https://doi.org/10.1007/978-3-030-41350-7_3

- If hernia sac not completely resected, significantly increased incidence of recurrence
- Use biologic mesh if you are going to use mesh
- Mesh has better short term outcomes, however no benefit has been shown in long-term outcomes
- Consider placing G-tube to tack stomach in abdomen

Patient Preparation

Supine with the surgeon on the right side of the patient and the assistant on the left.

If using a split leg table set-up, the surgeon stands between the patient's legs with the assistant to the left of the patient.

Anesthesia

General anesthesia.

Operative Steps

There may be some variations in port placement and choice of fundoplication based on patient specifics and surgeon choice. This section discusses one option.

1. A Veress needle is used to enter the abdomen at Palmer's point in the left upper quadrant and the abdomen is insufflated to 15 mmHg. Using a 0-degree camera, a 5 mm optical trocar is placed under direct vision at Palmer's point. Three additional 5 mm ports are placed in the upper abdomen along with a liver retractor placed through a subxiphoid incision. The camera is switched to a 5 mm 30-degree laparoscope.
2. The hiatus is visualized and as much of the paraesophageal hernia as possible is reduced back into the abdomen

using atraumatic graspers in a hand-over-hand pull of the stomach into the abdominal cavity.

3. The gastrohepatic ligament is divided with an energy device, exposing the right crus of the diaphragm.

4. The dissection along the diaphragmatic hiatus is continued superiorly and across to the left side, dissecting free the gastrophrenic ligament.

5. The dissection is continued posteriorly in the lesser sac to expose the junction of the right and left crura. Care should be taken to not injure the left gastric artery.

6. A penrose is passed in the retroesophageal space to allow adequate retraction of the gastroesophageal junction.

7. Care should be taken to avoid injury to the anterior/posterior vagus nerves, the aorta posteriorly and the inferior vena cava to the right of the diaphragmatic hiatus.

8. Complete circumferential mobilization, extending into the mediastinum is performed in order to obtain at least 3 cm of the distal esophagus in the abdominal cavity. Rarely, a gastroplasty will need to be performed to elongate the intra-abdominal esophagus.

9. At this time a bougie is passed through the mouth and into the esophagus. Care should be taken to avoid esophageal perforation.

10. The esophagus is retracted to the left upper quadrant by the assistant surgeon and the crus of the diaphragm is approximated posteriorly with interrupted nonabsorbable suture.

11. An antireflux procedure with either a Nissen fundoplication (360 degree wrap of the fundus of the stomach around the esophagus) or a Toupet fundoplication (270 degree posterior wrap of the fundus around the esophagus) is then performed.

12. The bougie is removed and an optional flexible endoscopy is performed to make sure the fundoplication is not too tight.

13. Laparoscopic ports are then removed and incisions are closed.

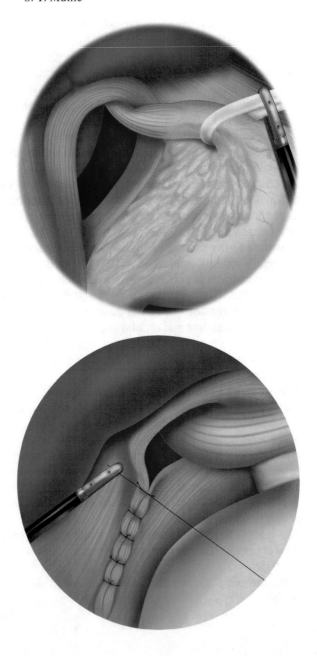

Chapter 4
Minimally Invasive Ivor Lewis Esophagectomy

Yasaman Kavousi

Overview

- Dissection through gastrohepatic ligament
- Identify right crus, and dissect posteriorly
- Divide gastrocolic ligament to enter lesser sac
- Mobilize stomach from pylorus to left crus, dividing short gastrics
- Preserve right gastroepiploic arcade, divide left gastroepiploic arcade
- Expose celiac axis and dissect nodal tissue
- Dissection continues cephalad to free esophagus
- Create gastric conduit using endostapler
- Create loop jejunostomy for feeding access
- Convert to thoracoscopic portion
- Take down inferior pulmonary ligament
- Mobilize esophagus from hiatus to thoracic inlet
- Azygous vein identified and divided
- Divide esophagus at carina, and bring conduit into chest, then esophagus divided proximally

Y. Kavousi (✉)
Department of General Surgery,
Henry Ford Hospital/Wayne State University, Detroit, MI, USA
e-mail: ykavousi@hfhs.org

© Springer Nature Switzerland AG 2020
E. Karamanos (ed.), *Common Surgeries Made Easy*,
https://doi.org/10.1007/978-3-030-41350-7_4

15

- Esophagogastrostomy created with stapler, then oversewn
- Chest tube placed

Clinical Pearls

- Replaced left hepatic artery courses through gastrohepatic ligament
- Right gastroepiploic is the vascular pedicle for neoesophagus

Patient Preparation

1. Abdominal portion: Supine with both arms out and footboard in place.
2. Thoracic portion: Left lateral decubitus with right arm extended over patient.

Preoperative foley placement and weight-based venous thromboembolism prophylaxis.

Anesthesia

General anesthesia via a double-lumen endotracheal tube.

Operative Steps

Abdominal Portion

1. An esophagogastroscopy is performed with a flexible endoscope to confirm the tumor location, and to assess the stomach's appropriateness to be used as a conduit.
2. With the patient in a supine position, the abdomen and lower chest are prepped and draped in the usual sterile fashion.

3. A 10 mm incision is then made to the left and superior to the umbilicus. The peritoneal cavity is then accessed using a Veress needle and pneumoperitoneum is established.

4. The intraperitoneal cavity is inspected for any evidence of metastatic disease using a 30-degree laparoscope.

5. Standard laparoscopic ports are then placed, including a self-retaining liver retractor.

6. Dissection is started by incising the gastrohepatic omentum to identify the right diaphragmatic crus.

7. The gastroesophageal junction is freed from the hiatus by dissecting up the right crus and extending the dissection to the left crus until the esophagus is dissected circumferentially from the mediastinum.

8. Using the Harmonic scalpel, the gastrocolic ligament is then divided lateral to the right gastroepiploic arcade to enter the lesser sac.

9. The greater curve of the stomach is then mobilized from the level of pylorus all the way to the left crus, taking down the short gastric arteries, with care taken to preserve the right gastroepiploic arcade.

10. The retroperitoneal attachments are taken down and the stomach is retracted superiorly and to the right to expose the celiac vessels. Any celiac and gastric nodal tissue is sent for pathology.

11. The left gastric artery is then isolated and divided using a vascular load of the EndoGIA stapler.

12. A penrose drain is then cut and placed around the esophagus to aid in retraction.

13. The right pleural space is then entered and the penrose drain is placed in the right pleural space to be retrieved during the thoracoscopic portion of the procedure.

14. The pylorus is then identified, and using an endostitch device, two 0-Ethibond stay sutures (superior and inferior) are placed along the horizontal axis of the pylorus to provide cephalad-caudal retraction. Two hundred units of botulinum toxin is then injected into the pylorus.

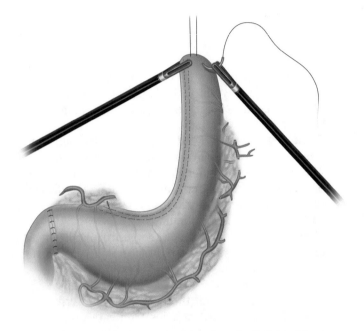

FIGURE 4.1 Creation of neo-esophagus based off of the right gastro-epiploic artery

15. The lesser omentum is then divided between the second and third vascular arcades using a vascular load of the EndoGIA stapler.
16. A 4–5 cm wide gastric conduit is then constructed by using a series of EndoGIA staple loads fired across the lesser curve. Gentle caudal retraction is applied to keep the conduit straight (Fig. 4.1).
17. The conduit is then tacked to the proximal stomach using two interrupted 0-Ethibond sutures.
18. Next, a feeding jejunostomy is created 30–40 cm distal to the ligament of Treitz.
19. All trocars are removed, and pneumoperitoneum is released. The port sites are closed with Dermabond and Steri-strips. A sterile dressing is applied.

Thoracic Portion

1. The patient is repositioned into the left lateral decubitus position.
2. The position of the double lumen endotracheal tube is confirmed and the right lung is isolated.
3. The right pleural space is accessed through an incision just anterior to the tip of the scapula in the 4th intercostal space.
4. CO_2 is insufflated to a pressure of 8 mmHg.
5. The camera is inserted and the thoracic cavity inspected for any intrapleural pathology.
6. The remaining standard robotic trocars are placed.
7. The robot is docked and the surgeon scrubs out to sit at the console. The assistant will remain scrubbed in.
8. The dissection begins by taking down the inferior pulmonary ligament using hook electrocautery.
9. Using electrocautery, the mediastinal pleura is dissected anteriorly along the plane between the esophagus and edge of the lung. In doing so, the esophagus is mobilized from the hiatus to the thoracic inlet.
10. The azygos vein is identified and divided using a vascular stapler.
11. Any aortic branches to the esophagus are identified and ligated with metallic clips.
12. Once the esophagus is satisfactorily mobilized, it is transected at the level of the carina using an EndoGIA stapler (Fig. 4.2).
13. The conduit is then delivered into the chest. The specimen is separated from the conduit by cutting the previously placed sutures.
14. The subcarinal lymph nodes are taken en bloc with the specimen and sent for pathology.
15. The specimen is removed in an EndoCatch bag by extending the assistant port incision by about 4–5 cm.
16. The specimen is examined on the back table to ensure wide proximal and distal margins.

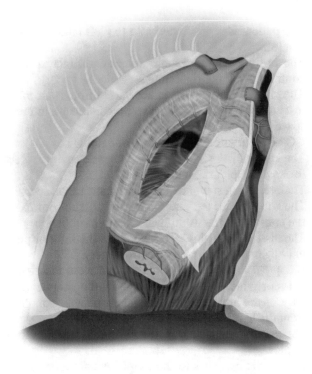

FIGURE 4.2 Thoracoscopic dissection of intrathoracic portion of the esophagus

17. The gastric conduit is gently grasped distally (to reduce tension), and then proximally by the staple line, and is positioned behind the esophagus immediately above the level of the azygos vein.
18. Indocyanine green is injected intravenously to assess perfusion of the conduit and esophagus, using Firefly® fluorescent imaging.
19. After confirmation of perfusion to the conduit, the esophagus is tacked to the conduit using four 2-0 silk sutures.
20. The EndoGIA stapler is used to create the back wall of the esophagogastric anastomosis.

21. The front wall of the anastomosis is done in two layers of interrupted 3-0 Vicryl followed by a running 3-0 Stratafix suture.
22. Prior to completion of the front wall, a nasogastric tube is inserted and placed through the conduit under direct vision.
23. The gastric staple line is over-sewn using a running 3-0 Stratafix suture (Fig. 4.3).
24. The robotic instruments are removed and the robot is undocked.
25. A 32-French chest tube is inserted through a separate incision, directed posteriorly toward the apex of the chest and attached to a pleur-evac.
26. The lung is re-inflated under direct vision.
27. All incisions are closed in layers using a 0-Vicryl suture followed by a 2-0 Vicryl suture. The skin is closed using a 4-0 Vicryl suture.
28. Just prior to extubation, the nasogastric tube is bridled using an umbilical tape.

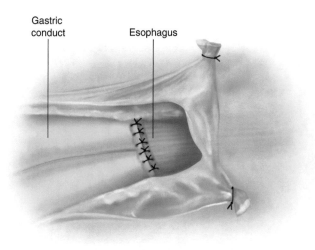

FIGURE 4.3 Completion of esophago - gastrostomy

Part II
Stomach

Chapter 5
The Graham Patch

Ryan Shelden

Overview

- Identify perforation, inspect proximal duodenum as well
- Mobilize omentum, to allow buttress at perforation site
- Using 2-0 silk sutures, take full thickness bites of healthy tissue at perforation
- Lay omentum over perforation, and tie sutures down gently

Clinical Pearls

- Patient can have delayed presentation due to ascites being sterile
- If on PPI preop, will need to perform vagotomy
- If perforation involves pylorus, can do pyloroplasty after debriding to healthy tissue
- Send tissue to pathology to rule out cancer, H. pylori

  - Gold standard for H. pylori identification is pathology

R. Shelden (✉)
Division of Acute Care Surgery and Critical Care,
Henry Ford Hospital/Wayne State University, Detroit, MI, USA

© Springer Nature Switzerland AG 2020
E. Karamanos (ed.), *Common Surgeries Made Easy*,
https://doi.org/10.1007/978-3-030-41350-7_5

- Modified Graham patch primarily close perforation and buttress omentum over top
- Consider UGI to rule out leak prior to removing NGT, and starting diet

Patient Preparation

Supine with both arms extended and footboard in place. Preoperative nasogastric tube placement. The surgeon stands on the left side of the patient with the assistant on the patient's right side.

Anesthesia

General anesthesia.

Operative Steps

1. A vertical midline incision is made in the epigastric region.
2. The fascia is opened and development of the preperitoneal space is aided by digital dissection. The peritoneum is grasped with hemostats, lifted anteriorly, and sharply divided with Metzenbaum scissors.
3. Aerobic and anaerobic cultures are sent to pathology from the peritoneal fluid.
4. The stomach is exposed and inspected for perforation. The left lobe of the liver is elevated to inspect the proximal duodenum. If the perforation remains elusive, the anesthesiologist may assist by insufflating the stomach via the nasogastric tube.
5. If the perforation is prepyloric or duodenal and suitable for a Graham patch, the omentum is identified via its attachment to the transverse colon and a well-vascularized mobile pedicle that reaches the perforation without any tension is developed.

6. Three to four interrupted full-thickness 2-0 silk sutures are placed across the defect in a fashion that is parallel to the axis of the viscera.
7. The omental pedicle is placed over the defect between the tails of the sutures, which are tied over the omentum without strangulation of the pedicle (Fig. 5.1).
8. A thorough lavage of the abdomen is performed, paying particular attention to the bilateral paracolic and subphrenic recesses.
9. The decision to place drains depends on surgeon's preference.
10. The abdominal fascia is closed with a continuous #1 PDS.
11. The subcutaneous tissue is irrigated and may be loosely closed or left open to heal by secondary intention.

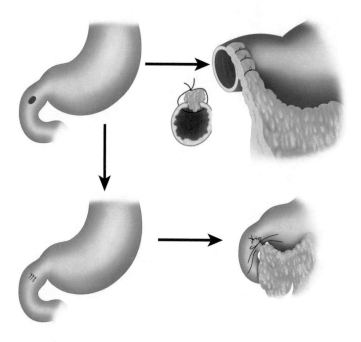

FIGURE 5.1 The tongue of omentum acts as a plug for the perforation. The original Graham patch does not include primary closure of the defect

Chapter 6
Billroth 1 Gastroduodenostomy

Tommy Ivanics and Rupen Shah

Overview

- Open the lesser sac via the gastrocolic ligament
- Dissect distally towards the duodenum on the greater curvature of the stomach
- Perform a Kocher maneuver, and then dissect circumferentially
- Open the gastrohepatic ligament, and dissect along lesser curve of stomach
- Perform vagotomy if indicated
- Transect the duodenum at D2, then staple across the stomach to remove the specimen
- Perform a gastroduodenostomy

T. Ivanics (✉)
Department of General Surgery, Henry Ford Hospital/Wayne State University, Detroit, MI, USA
e-mail: tivanic1@hfhs.org

R. Shah
Division of Surgical Oncology, Department of Surgery, Henry Ford Hospital/Wayne State University, Detroit, MI, USA

© Springer Nature Switzerland AG 2020
E. Karamanos (ed.), *Common Surgeries Made Easy*,
https://doi.org/10.1007/978-3-030-41350-7_6

Clinical Pearls

- The replaced left hepatic artery will run through the gastrohepatic ligament
- If too much tension is encountered after the D2 has been fully mobilized; perform a Billroth II
- Pay attention to the angle of Sorrow → close with triple seromuscular stitch
- Extent of the full Kocher maneuver: Inferior to the right renal vein, superior to the portal vein, medial to pancreatic head
- Dumping syndrome can occur postoperatively → if intractable convert to Roux-en-Y
    - Type 1: hyperosmotic load causing fluid shift into the bowel resulting in hypotension, diarrhea, dizziness
    - Type 2: hypoglycemia from increased insulin and decreased glucose
- Alkaline reflux syndrome can also occur → if intractable convert to Roux-en-Y

Patient Preparation

Supine with arms out. Prep skin with chloraprep and place a foley catheter.

Antibiotic and venous thromboembolism prophylaxis, and placement of a nasogastric tube.

Anesthesia

General anesthesia with or without epidural catheter placement.

Operative Considerations

The addition of a selective vagotomy of the gastric remnant for benign ulcer surgery is necessary only when gastric hypersecretion is the main pathogenetic factor (such as with multiple ulcers or prepyloric ulcers). This is accomplished by dividing the anterior and posterior vagal branches and sparing the hepatic vagal branches.

Operative Steps

1. Perform an upper midline incision from the xiphoid process to just below the umbilicus. Deepen the incision through the subcutaneous tissues and identify the linea alba, which is incised to enter the peritoneal cavity.
2. Using moistened laparotomy pads, pack the small bowel and colon inferiorly, and use retractors to hold them in place. This will allow for adequate exposure of the stomach and duodenum.
3. Perform a thorough abdominal exploration to identify the pathology in question (ulcer). Examine the pancreas and gallbladder by gentle palpation and identify any other pathologies such as gallstones.
4. Incise the gastrocolic ligament at the midpoint of the greater curve of the stomach. This will open the omental bursa.
5. Create an opening in the lesser omentum/gastrohepatic ligament and place a soft rubber Penrose drain around the stomach for retraction.
6. Dissect along the greater curve towards the duodenum and sequentially clamp and divide the gastroepiploic vessels using 2-0 silk ties.
7. Near the pylorus, the greater curve of the omentum splits into an anterior and posterior layer. Continue the dissection toward the duodenum and ligate any vessels individually.

8. Perform a Kocher maneuver. Do this by sharply cutting along the lateral duodenal wall from the second portion of the duodenum to the beginning of the hepatoduodenal ligament. Retract the second portion of the duodenum medially and loosen the retroperitoneal tissues through a combination of blunt and sharp dissection

9. Retract the stomach toward the left and superior direction. This will allow circumferential duodenal mobilization (proceeding from the left medial duodenal wall, then posteriorly to the back wall, and then laterally to the lateral duodenal wall to the level of the hepatoduodenal ligament). This typically exposes about 3–5 cm of the back wall of the duodenum.

10. Identify and protect the gastroduodenal artery. It can be identified at the transition point between the first free part of the duodenum and the fixed dorsal part where the serosa passes from the duodenum to the head of the pancreas.

11. Turn your attention to the lesser curve of the stomach to continue the dissection. Divide the right gastric artery between clamps and ligate using silk ties.

12. Optional: Perform a selective vagotomy of the remaining stomach only in cases of benign gastric ulcer surgery where the main pathogenetic factor is gastric acid hypersecretion (i.e., in cases of multiple ulcers or ulcers in a prepyloric location). Divide the vagal branches of the anterior and posterior vagus leading to the gastric remnant while leaving the hepatic branches intact.

13. Place stay/holding sutures on the lateral aspect of the duodenum, apply bowel clamps across the duodenum and sharply transect. Close the duodenum temporarily with a sponge.

14. Transect the stomach by using a stapler, either a TA90 stapling device (Covidien) or a TL90 (Ethicon), across the proximal resection margin at a 45-degree angle to the lesser curve. The staple line can be oversewn, but this is not mandatory. Hand off the specimen.

15. Place the duodenum and the greater curvature adjacent to each other. Place two corner stitches, starting on the outside and going inside, on the stomach side and inside going outside on the duodenum. Tie the corner suture at the lesser curvature but leave the suture on the opposite side untied.

16. Place a posterior row of interrupted, full-thickness stitches using 3-0 polyglycolic acid. The suture is then led back from inside the duodenum catching only the mucosa first on the duodenum and then subsequently on the stomach, ending on the inside of the stomach portion.

17. Close the front wall with one row of an interrupted seromuscular suture with tangential grabbing of the mucosa similar to the initial corner stitches.

18. Pay careful attention to the Jammerecke (angle of Sorrow) on the lesser curvature. This can be closed using a triple seromuscular suture, including the duodenal walls and front and back wall of the stomach. Alternatively, a seromuscular stitch can be taken outside going inside on the front wall of the stomach, followed by a seromuscular bite of the duodenum and then a seromuscular bite of the back wall of the stomach ending on the outside.

19. Place a nasogastric gastric tube across the anastomosis.

20. Secure the vascular pedicles to the ligated gastric pedicles of the duodenum with 4-0 silk sutures and cover the repair with omentum.

21. Close the abdominal fascia using running #1 PDS suture with 5 mm travel and 5 mm bites.

22. Close the subcutaneous tissues and Camper's fascia with an interrupted 3-0 Vicryl stitch.

23. Close the skin with a running subcuticular 4-0 monocryl stitch.

Chapter 7
Billroth 2 Gastroenterostomy

Tommy Ivanics and Rupen Shah

Overview

- Open the lesser sac via the gastrocolic ligament, and dissect the greater curve of the stomach toward the duodenum
- Perform a Kocher maneuver, and then dissect circumferentially
- Open the gastrohepatic ligament, and dissect the lesser curve of the stomach
- Perform a vagotomy if indicated
- Transect the duodenum at D2, then staple across the stomach to remove the specimen
- Bring the jejunum retrocolic, and perform a gastrojejunostomy

T. Ivanics (✉)
Department of General Surgery, Henry Ford Hospital/Wayne State University, Detroit, MI, USA
e-mail: tivanic1@hfhs.org

R. Shah
Division of Surgical Oncology, Department of Surgery, Henry Ford Hospital/Wayne State University, Detroit, MI, USA

© Springer Nature Switzerland AG 2020
E. Karamanos (ed.), *Common Surgeries Made Easy*,
https://doi.org/10.1007/978-3-030-41350-7_7

Clinical Pearls

- Extent of a Full Kocher maneuver: Inferior to the right renal vein, superior to the portal vein, medial to the pancreatic head
- Dumping syndrome → if intractable convert to Roux-en-Y
  - Type 1: hyperosmotic load causing fluid shift into bowel resulting in hypotension, diarrhea, dizziness
  - Type 2: hypoglycemia from increased insulin and decreased glucose

- Alkaline reflux syndrome → if intractable convert to Roux-en-Y with afferent limb 60 cm distal to gastrojejunostomy

  - will have bile in stomach and gastritis on EGD

- Blind loop syndrome treat medically → if refractory reanastamose with shorter afferent limb

  - caused by poor motility and bacterial overgrowth
- Afferent loop syndrome → can balloon dilate or reanastamose with shorter afferent limb

  - caused by mechanical obstruction of the afferent limb

Patient Preparation

Supine with arms out. Prep skin with chloraprep and place a foley catheter.

Antibiotic prophylaxis, nasogastric tube, venous thromboembolism prophylaxis.

Anesthesia

General anesthesia with or without an epidural catheter placed preoperatively.

Operative Considerations

The addition of a selective vagotomy of the gastric remnant for benign ulcer surgery is necessary only where gastric hypersecretion is the main pathogenetic factor (such as with multiple ulcers or prepyloric ulcers). This is accomplished by the division of the anterior and posterior vagal branches with sparing of the hepatic vagal branches.

Operative Steps

1. Perform an upper midline incision from the xiphoid process to just below umbilicus, similar to a Billroth 1.
2. Deepen the incision through subcutaneous tissues and identify the linea alba, incise, and enter the peritoneal cavity.
3. Place a self-retaining retractor and with moistened laparotomy pads, pack the small bowel, and colon inferiorly. This will allow for adequate exposure of the stomach and duodenum.
4. Explore the abdominal cavity for pathology and adhesions. Examine the pancreas and the gallbladder by gentle palpation.
5. Incise the gastrocolic ligament at the midpoint of the greater curvature of the stomach. This will open the omental bursa.
6. Create an opening in the lesser sac/gastrohepatic ligament and place a flexible rubber drain circumferentially around the stomach to facilitate retraction.
7. Continue the dissection along the greater curvature toward the duodenum and clamp, divide and ligate the gastroepiploic vessels using 2-0 silk ties or with a ligasure device.
8. Near the pylorus, the greater curvature of the omentum splits into an anterior and posterior layer, carry the dissection between these layers toward the duodenum and ligate any vessels individually.

9. Once the duodenum is reached, perform a Kocher maneuver. Do this by sharply cutting along the lateral duodenal wall from the second portion of the duodenum to the beginning of the hepatoduodenal ligament. Retract the second portion of the duodenum medially and loosen the retroperitoneal tissues with a combination of blunt and sharp dissection.

10. Retract the stomach in a leftward and superior direction. This will allow circumferential duodenal mobilization (proceeding from the left medial duodenal wall, posteriorly to the back wall, and then laterally to the lateral duodenal wall to the level of the hepatoduodenal ligament). This typically exposes about 3–5 cm of the back wall of the duodenum.

11. Identify and protect the gastroduodenal artery. It can be identified at the transition point between the first free part of the duodenum and the fixed dorsal part where the serosa passes from the duodenum to the head of the pancreas.

12. Divide the duodenum with a linear stapler, a TA-55 (Covidien), or a TL60 (Ethicon), 2 cm distal to the pylorus.

13. Oversew the duodenal stump with seromuscular interrupted sutures using a resorbable 3-0 suture.

14. Close the antrum temporarily using a clamp.

15. Continue the dissection along the greater curve to within 3–4 cm of the esophagus. Divide the right gastric artery between clamps and ligate using silk ties.

16. Preserve the left gastric and left gastroepiploic arteries.

17. At the proximal dissection line, complete the transection using a linear stapler (TA-90) so that the entire stomach is divided using one staple load.

18. Optional: Perform a selective vagotomy of the remaining stomach only in cases of benign gastric ulcer disease where the main pathogenetic factor is gastric acid hypersecretion (i.e., in cases of multiple ulcers or ulcers in a prepyloric location). Divide the vagal branches of the anterior and posterior vagus leading to the gastric remnant while leaving the hepatic branches intact.

19. Mobilize the first or second loop of jejunum and place the jejunal loop in a retrocolic fashion opposite the greater curvature of the remnant stomach, ensuring that there is no tension. Ensure that the loop is long enough to accommodate a Braun enterostomy (jejunojejunostomy) between the ascending and the descending limb.

20. Excise the last 4–5 cm of the staple line toward the greater curve using electrocautery to create a small opening for the gastrojejunostomy.

21. Ensure adequate hemostasis of the front and back wall of the stomach.

22. Incise the jejunum with electrocautery on the antimesenteric surface.

23. Create the gastrojejunostomy with a single interrupted suture with resorbable 3-0 suture. Suture the back wall using interrupted mattress sutures and the front wall by extramucosal interrupted sutures. Alternatively, the anastomosis can be performed by a continuous suture using a resorbable 3-0 monofilament on the front and back wall of the anastomosis (Fig. 7.1).

    Alternatively, a two-layered anastomosis can be performed with an inner layer of a running 3-0 Vicryl suture followed by an outer layer of interrupted 3-0 silk Lembert sutures. Ensure that a three-point suture is placed at the angle of sorrow.

    If stapled: Approximate the jejunum to the posterior wall of the stomach using two sutures of 3-0 silk sutures. Create a gastrotomy and a jejunostomy and insert a linear stapler and fire it. Inspect the staple line for hemostasis. Close the enterotomies with a linear stapler or in two layers using 3-0 Vicryl sutures followed by 3-0 silk sutures (Fig. 7.1).

24. Before completing the anastomosis, pass a double-lumen gastric tube distal to the anastomosis to allow early enteral nutrition.

25. Create a Braun enterostomy (jejunojejunostomy) in a side-to-side fashion 30 cm distal to the gastrojejunostomy. This is performed to prevent bile reflux. Perform this either handsewn (interrupted or running 3-0 suture) or by using a stapler.

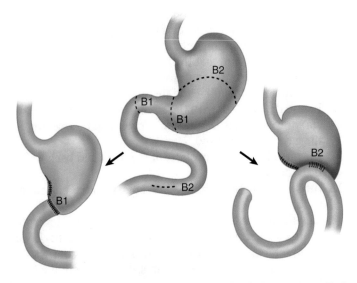

Figure 7.1 Gastric reconstruction after distal gastrectomy. Left depicts an end to end gastroduodenostomy (Billroth 1). On the right, an end to side gastrojejunostomy is depicted (Billroth 2)

26. Cover the repair with omentum.
27. Close the abdominal fascia using a running #1 PDS suture with 5 mm travel and 5 mm bites.
28. Close the subcutaneous tissues and the Camper's fascia with an interrupted 3-0 Vicryl sutures.
29. Close the skin with a running 4-0 subcuticular Vicryl stitch.

Chapter 8
Subtotal Gastrectomy with D2 Lymphadenectomy

Tommy Ivanics and Rupen Shah

Overview

- Greater curve mobilization, greater omentectomy, left gastroepiploic vessels division
- Infrapyloric mobilization, right gastroepiploic vessel ligation
- Suprapyloric mobilization, right gastric vessels ligation
- Duodenal transection
- D2 lymphadenectomy, dissection of PH, CHA, LGA, CA, SA, left gastric vessel ligation
- Gastric transection
- Loop or Roux-en-y gastrojejunostomy reconstruction

T. Ivanics (✉)
Department of General Surgery, Henry Ford Hospital/Wayne State University, Detroit, MI, USA
e-mail: tivanic1@hfhs.org

R. Shah
Division of Surgical Oncology, Department of Surgery, Henry Ford Hospital/Wayne State University, Detroit, MI, USA

© Springer Nature Switzerland AG 2020   41
E. Karamanos (ed.), *Common Surgeries Made Easy*,
https://doi.org/10.1007/978-3-030-41350-7_8

Clinical Pearls

- If performing a concomitant splenectomy, do not perform a high ligation of the left gastric artery, as this will cause gastric remnant necrosis
- Crow's foot courses over the pylorus, so dissection distal to this includes the entire stomach
- Duodenum has Brunner's glands which secrete HCO3; if absent on pathology, dissection is incomplete

Preoperative Considerations

A careful cancer workup with consideration for a staging laparoscopy (25% of patients are upstaged, this procedure allows for placement of a feeding jejunostomy tube) and preoperative systemic therapy.

Patient Preparation

Supine with arms out. Prep skin with chloraprep and place a foley catheter and nasogastric tube.

Preoperative antibiotics (second-generation cephalosporin), venous thromboembolism prophylaxis.

Anesthesia

General, with or without an epidural catheter placed preoperatively.

Operative Considerations

Need a 5 cm margin from the tumor, and at least 15 lymph nodes sampled. Perform a total gastrectomy when 5–6 cm of negative margins cannot be achieved from the primary tumor.

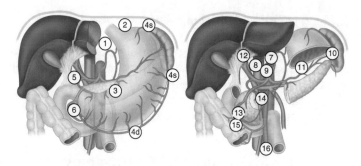

FIGURE 8.1   Lymph node stations

Lymphadenectomy

D1: Perigastric nodes (station 1–6)

D2: Lymph nodes along the common hepatic, left gastric, splenic arteries (stations 7–11)

D3: Additional nodes within the porta hepatis and adjacent to the aorta (stations 12–16) (Fig. 8.1)

Nodal Dissection

Three potential purposes: 1. Staging 2. Prevention of locoregional recurrence 3. Improvement in overall survival.

Distal/subtotal gastrectomy: D1 (1, 3, 4sb, 4d, 5, 6, 7) + 8a, 9, 11p, 12a

Proximal gastrectomy: N/A

Total gastrectomy: D1 (1–7) + 8a, 9,10, 11p, 11d, 12a

Operative Steps: D2 for Subtotal/Distal Gastrectomy

1. Greater curve mobilization, greater omentectomy, left gastroepiploic vessel division
2. Infrapyloric mobilization, right gastroepiploic vessel ligation

3. Suprapyloric mobilization, right gastric vessel ligation
4. Duodenal transection
5. D2 lymphadenectomy, dissection of porta hepatis, common hepatic artery, left gastric artery, celiac trunk, splenic artery, left gastric vessel ligation
6. Gastric transection
7. Loop or Roux-en-y gastrojejunostomy reconstruction

Operative Steps: Subtotal Gastrectomy with D2 Lymphadenectomy, Greater Curvature (Station 4sb and 4d) Node Dissection

1. Perform a diagnostic laparoscopy to exclude distant disease such as liver and peritoneal metastases, or remote lymph node involvement, which all preclude resection. Obtain a wash cytology in the upper abdomen.
2. Perform a midline laparotomy from the xiphoid to just below the umbilicus.
3. Deepen the incision through the subcutaneous tissues, and identify the linea alba, incise and enter the peritoneal cavity.
4. Divide the falciform ligament and place a self-retaining retractor (such as a Thompson or Bookwalter) on the abdominal wall.
5. Assess the primary tumor for the proximal and the distal extent and any possible locoregional invasion. A marking suture may be placed on the anterior gastric wall to mark the proximal extent of the tumor.
6. Dissect the greater omentum off the transverse colon using electrocautery, beginning from the center and moving to the left. The dissection should be bloodless if performed in the correct avascular plane between the omentum and the epiploic appendages of the colon.
7. Reflect the greater omentum superiorly.
8. Continue the dissection on the left side of the abdomen so that the greater omentum is taken off the splenic flex-

ure and the inferior pole of the spleen. This should expose the body and tail of the pancreas.

9. Divide the left gastroepiploic vessels near their origin from the splenic vessels just anterior to the pancreas.

10. Elevate the spleen into the operative field with moist lap pads placed posteriorly. Lyse omental and colonic attachments to the spleen if needed to avoid inadvertent capsular tears during the dissection.

11. *For a distal subtotal gastrectomy, the short gastric vessels must be preserved as the other arteries supplying the gastric remnant are divided.*

12. Identify the greater curvature of the stomach between the end of the left gastroepiploic arcade and the start of the short gastric vessels. This marks the leftmost extent of the greater omentum dissection.

13. Divide the omentum from peripherally toward the gastric wall. Once the gastric wall is reached, use ultrasonic coagulating shears to dissect between the gastric wall and greater omentum from proximal to distal.

Infrapyloric (station 6) node dissection, mobilization

14. Once a full mobilization of the left side of the stomach has been achieved, continue the dissection of the omentum toward the hepatic flexure of the colon.

15. Identify the colic branch of the gastrocolic trunk within the transverse mesocolon. Follow it to its confluence with the right gastroepiploic vein, which forms the short gastrocolic trunk. The trunk drains to the superior mesenteric vein.

16. *For distal stomach tumors, the nodal tissue anterior, medial and lateral to the superior mesenteric vein at the inferior portion of the pancreas, station 14, should be resected and sent off separately.*

17. Dissect the infrapyloric lymph nodes off the head of the pancreas. Proceed cautiously in this area to avoid tearing small vessels which may lead to troublesome bleeding. This may be facilitated by the use of ultrasonic coagulating shears.

18. Sweep all the soft tissues anterior to the pancreas superiorly onto the specimen.
19. Identify the right gastroepiploic vein at its origin from the inferior pancreaticoduodenal arcade. It is ligated and divided at its juncture with the gastrocolic trunk and the inferior pancreaticoduodenal arcade.
20. Identify the right gastroepiploic artery and divide it at its origin from the gastroduodenal artery.
21. Dissect the station 6 lymph nodes off the head of the pancreas and include them in the specimen.
22. Create a tunnel/plane between the first portion of the duodenum and the head of the pancreas. Sweep all nodal and soft tissue off the pancreas and onto the specimen.

Hepatoduodenal ligament, Hepatic Artery (Station 12a) and suprapyloric (station 5) node dissection.

23. Divide the gastrohepatic ligament, taking care to identify an accessory or replaced left hepatic artery if one is present. If a replaced/accessory left hepatic artery is identified it may be divided unless the patient has underlying liver dysfunction.
24. Open the hepatoduodenal ligament vertically in the direction of the proper hepatic artery, completely exposing the right gastric and gastroduodenal arteries. This should be done from the mid lesser omentum near the undersurface of the liver towards the superior porta hepatis.
25. Dissect this nodal tissue from the right or left, which should allow complete exposure of the common hepatic artery/proper hepatic artery/gastroduodenal artery trifurcation.
26. Dissect on the lateral border of the proper hepatic artery from superior to inferior.
27. Divide the soft tissue between the suprapyloric nodes and the proper hepatic artery nodes.
28. Carry the dissection posteriorly to the left of the proper hepatic artery to expose the left side of the portal vein.
29. Divide the right gastric artery at its origin from either the proper hepatic artery or the gastroduodenal artery using 2-0 silk ties.

30. Dissect the station 5 lymph nodes with the specimen.
31. Ligate any small vessels and take down any residual fatty attachments to allow full mobilization of the duodenum.
32. Develop the plane between the superior first portion of the duodenum and the underlying pancreas until the prior dissection from inferiorly is reached.
33. Ligate small vessels to the first portion of the duodenum with a harmonic sealing device. This effectively will mobilize the entire 1st portion of the duodenum.

<u>Duodenal transection</u>

34. Transect the duodenum 1 cm distal to the pylorus (unless tumor invasion of the duodenum is suspected which would require a more distal resection margin) using a GIA stapler blue load
35. Place interrupted 3-0 silk Lembert sutures on the staple line to achieve inversion of the duodenal stump.

<u>Common hepatic artery dissection (station 8a), Celiac axis (station 9), proximal splenic artery (station 11p), and left gastric artery (station 7) lymph node dissection; D2 Lymphadenectomy</u>

36. Divide the peritoneum and lymphatics in the superior porta hepatis from the right to left until the lesser omentum opening is reached.
37. Dissect off the nodal tissue of the lateral aspect of the proper hepatic artery toward the left side of the abdomen.
38. Gently retract the proper hepatic artery to the right side of the abdomen and dissect free the nodal tissue along the anterior surface of the portal vein and the posterior surface of the proper hepatic artery.
39. The station 12 lymph nodes and the investing fibrofatty connective tissue are pulled into the omental bursa to the left of the porta hepatis.
40. Continue the dissection along the superior border of the pancreas, and divide tissue between the common hepatic artery and pancreas and include this tissue with the station 8 lymph nodes along with the anterior and the poste-

rior aspects of the common hepatic artery. Due to the vascularity of this nodal tissue a harmonic scalpel is recommended during this dissection.

41. Identify the left gastric, or coronary vein which courses posteriorly from the lesser curvature. Ligate and divide it at its confluence with the portal or splenic vein.

42. Dissect free the nodal tissue at the upper border of the pancreas along with proximal splenic artery (station 11). Sweep it superiorly and to the left together with the other lymphatic tissue.

43. Continue the dissection medially to the celiac axis. Skeletonize the celiac artery and its branches. Identify the left gastric artery and suture ligate it at its origin. Adjacent nodal tissue is reflected toward the crura of the diaphragm.

44. Proceed dissecting proximally along the lesser curve of the stomach to the right border of the esophagus.

45. Free the peritoneum overlying the anterior surface of the abdominal esophagus.

46. Dissect the nodal tissue along the right cardia (station 1) off the GEJ and the anterior wall of the lesser curvature of the stomach.

47. Ensure that the dissection is carried proximal along the lesser curve (beyond the level of the planned level of transection), which may include 2–3 cm of the intra-abdominal esophagus, as the left gastric artery usually bifurcates high on the lesser curve (frequently at the level of the GEJ) into superior and inferior branches.

48. Continue the nodal dissection along the splenic artery to the posterior gastric artery which arises from the splenic artery and supplies the posteromedial wall of the stomach. Clear all nodal tissue anterior and superior to the proximal splenic artery until retroperitoneal fat is encountered.

49. *The dissection does not routinely need to extend into the splenic hilum (station 10) unless gross involvement is apparent. Splenectomy is performed only for locoregional disease and does not need to be performed routinely for a*

D2 lymphadenectomy due to the associated increase in morbidity without survival benefit

Gastric transection

50. Identify a line which connects a point approximately 2 cm distal to the GEJ on the lesser curvature and a point at least 5 cm proximal to the upper border of the tumor on the greater curvature of the stomach.
51. Place straight bowel clamps on the greater curvature for a distance of approximately 6–8 cm.
52. Divide the stomach between these clamps with a knife.
53. The remaining stomach from the tips of the straight clamps to the chosen point on the lesser curve is divided with the GIA stapler to create a short Hofmeister shelf. Send the proximal and distal margins for frozen section analysis. Send the proximal and distal margins for frozen section analysis.
54. Invert the staple line with a running monofilament suture.
55. Pass off the specimen and label the relevant lymph node groups for pathology assessment.

Reconstruction

56. Choose one of two reconstructions: a Billroth II loop gastrojejunostomy or a Roux-en-Y gastrojejunostomy.
57. If a Billroth II loop gastrojejunostomy is chosen: choose a loop of jejunum just distal to the ligament of Treitz and bring it to the gastric pouch either in an antecolic or a retrocolic fashion (in relation to the transverse colon). Ensure that no tension or angulation is present. Avoid an excessively long limb as this may lead to development of afferent loop syndrome.
58. Bring the jejunal loop to the gastric pouch in a side-to-side isoperistaltic fashion with the proximal end of the jejunum apposed to the lesser curve of the stomach opening.
59. Place an outer, posterior row of interrupted 3-0 silk seromuscular (Lembert) sutures between the posterior gastric wall and the jejunum.

60. Remove the straight clamp from the stomach and make an incision in the jejunum just slightly shorter than the gastrotomy using electrocautery.
61. Create the inner, posterior layer of the anastomosis with a running 3-0 PDS suture in a simple over-and-over fashion, including the full thickness of both the stomach and the jejunal walls.
62. Continue the inner layer anastomosis anteriorly as a running Connell suture, which will cause an anastomotic inversion.
63. Advance the nasogastric tube through the gastric remnant into the efferent jejunal limb prior to the completion of the anastomosis.
64. Complete the anterior portion of the gastrojejunostomy with interrupted 3-0 silk lambert sutures.
65. Take special care during the placement of the three-cornered Lembert suture at the junction of the lesser curvature gastric staple line and the gastrojejunostomy; this is known as the angle of death.
66. *If a Roux-en-Y reconstruction is chosen:* Divide the jejunum approximately 20 cm distal to the ligament of Treitz and bring it up to the stomach through a defect to the left of the middle colic vessels in the transverse mesocolon.
67. Perform the gastrojejunal anastomosis in a fashion as previously described for the loop anastomosis.
68. Restore the intestinal continuity with a side-to-side jejunojejunostomy at least 50–60 cm distal to the gastrojejunostomy to prevent biliopancreatic reflex into the gastric remnant. The jejunojejunostomy may be performed either stapled or hand-sewn.
69. *If stapled:* Perform two small enterotomies in the antimesenteric borders of the small intestine. One fork of the GIA stapler is placed in each of the intestinal lumen and then fired.
70. The common enterotomy is closed either with a TA stapling device or a full thickness running monofilament suture after staple line hemostasis inspection
71. Ensure adequate hemostasis.

72. Close the fascia with a running suture of #1 PDS with a 5 mm travel and a 5 mm bite.
73. Close the Camper's fascia with an interrupted 3-0 Vicryl suture.
74. Close the skin using a 4-0 Vicryl suture in a subcuticular fashion.

Chapter 9
Total Gastrectomy

Tommy Ivanics and Rupen Shah

Overview

- Greater curve mobilization, greater omentectomy, left gastroepiploic vessels division
- Infrapyloric mobilization, right gastroepiploic vessel ligation
- Divide the short gastric arteries and bring all tissue with the specimen
- Incise the gastrohepatic ligament and identify and ligate the right gastric vessels, continue mobilization to the GEJ at the right crus
- Duodenal transection; include all nodal tissue with specimen
- Identify the left crus and keep all perinodal tissue with specimen
- D2 lymphadenectomy, dissection of PH, CHA, LGA, CA, SA, left gastric vessel ligation

T. Ivanics (✉)
Department of General Surgery, Henry Ford Hospital/Wayne State University, Detroit, MI, USA
e-mail: tivanic1@hfhs.org

R. Shah
Division of Surgical Oncology, Department of Surgery, Henry Ford Hospital/Wayne State University, Detroit, MI, USA

© Springer Nature Switzerland AG 2020
E. Karamanos (ed.), *Common Surgeries Made Easy*,
https://doi.org/10.1007/978-3-030-41350-7_9

53

- Gastric transection
- Esophagojejunostomy creation
- Roux-en-Y reconstruction
- Feeding jejunostomy tube insertion

Clinical Pearls

- Crow's foot courses over pylorus, so dissection distal to this includes entire stomach
- Duodenum has Brunner's glands which secrete HCO_3; if absent on pathology, dissection is incomplete

Nodal Dissection

Must sample at least 16 nodes

Three potential purposes: (1) Staging. (2) Prevention of locoregional recurrence. (3) Improvement in overall survival. The current recommendation is that at least 16 lymph nodes are examined for correct assessment of the N.

Distal/subtotal gastrectomy D1 (1, 3, 4sb, 4d, 5, 6, 7) +8a, 9, 11p, 12a

Proximal gastrectomy N/A

Total gastrectomy: D1 (1–7) + 8a, 9, 10, 11p, 11d, 12a

Patient Preparation

Supine with arms out. Prep abdomen with chloraprep, include the chest for proximal tumors that may require a combined thoracic approach, and place a foley catheter and nasogastric tube.

Sandbag under left costal margin.

Preoperative antibiotics (second generation cephalosporin).

Consider a staging laparoscopy (25% of patients are upstaged, this procedure allows for placement of feeding jejunostomy tube prior to preoperative systemic therapy).

Anesthesia

General with or without an epidural catheter placed preoperatively.

Operative Considerations

Need a 5–6 cm margin from tumor and at least 15 lymph nodes sampled.

Lymphadenectomy

D1: Perigastric nodes (station 1–6)
   D2: Lymph nodes along the common hepatic, left gastric, and splenic arteries (stations 7–11)
   D3: Additional nodes within the porta hepatis and adjacent to the aorta (stations 12–16)

Operative Steps: Total Gastrectomy with D2 Lymphadenectomy

1. Perform a diagnostic laparoscopy to exclude distant disease such as liver and peritoneal metastases and remote lymph node involvement, which will preclude resection. Obtain a peritoneal wash for cytology in the upper abdomen.
2. Perform a midline laparotomy from the xiphoid to just below the umbilicus.
3. Deepen the incision through the subcutaneous tissues and identify the linea alba, incise and enter the peritoneal cavity.
4. Place retractors to aid with exposure. Dissect the greater omentum from the colon using electrocautery, entering into the anterior leaflet of the mesocolon. Bleeding should be minimal if the correct plane is entered.
5. Mobilize the splenic flexure of the colon inferiorly.

6. Continue the dissection to the inferior border of the pancreas and dissect the pancreatic capsule cephalad.

7. Divide any branches of the right gastroepiploic vessels at the inferior border of the pancreas and carefully divide any venous tributaries. Ligate the right gastroepiploic vein just proximal to the insertion of the accessory right colic vein with 3-0 silk ligatures. Identify and ligate the right gastroepiploic artery with 3-0 silk ligatures.

8. Extend the dissection laterally along the superior portion of the pancreas, skeletonizing the splenic artery and dividing short gastric vessels close to the spleen. Leave the pancreatic capsule in situ to prevent a pancreatic leak. Separate all subpyloric lymphatic tissue from the duodenal wall and keep with the specimen.

9. Incise the peritoneum on the left side of the hepatoduodenal ligament and expose the right gastric artery. Ligate the artery using 2-0 silk ties and divide.

10. Dissect the lesser omentum from the inferior portion of the liver to the right crus of the diaphragm and the right aspect of the gastroesophageal junction. Include the nodal tissue in the specimen.

11. Place two straight Kocher clamps on the duodenum and divide using a GIA stapler (blue load) 1 cm distal to the pylorus. Reinforce the duodenal staple line with interrupted horizontal 3-0 monofilament absorbable mattress sutures.

12. Reflect the stomach cephalad, exposing the pancreas, common hepatic artery and the celiac axis. Begin the portal dissection by isolating the hepatic artery bifurcation, sweeping nodal tissue downward. Dissect the portal vein to the left of the left hepatic artery and in the area between the common hepatic and the superior border of the pancreas. Sweep this dissection back to the celiac axis and meet the dissection of the superior border of the pancreas at the junction of the splenic artery with the celiac.

13. Identify and divide the left gastric artery at its origin.

14. Dissect along the right crus to identify the celiac axis and clear off the nodal tissue.

15. The nodal tissue overlying the splenic artery should be dissected from the splenic hilum toward the left gastric artery. A splenectomy has no benefit unless it is performed for primary tumor clearance.

16. Identify the origin of the left gastroepiploic artery from the splenic artery and ligate. Identify and ligate any short gastric vessels close to the spleen, allowing for the identification of the left crus. Identify and preserve the left adrenal gland.

17. Once the entire stomach is mobilized, lift the entire stomach complex forward.

18. Dissect the left paracardial nodes by dividing the phreno-esophageal ligament and reflect the paracardial lymph nodes inferiorly with the specimen.

19. Mobilize the gastroesophageal junction with sharp and blunt dissection and encircle the esophagus with a Penrose drain. Identify the anterior and posterior vagus nerves, ligate and divide them.

20. Place a soft Satinsky atraumatic vascular clamp on the esophagus and transect using an endoscopic linear stapler (3.5 mm staple size).

21. Send the proximal margin for frozen section.

22. Identify the ligament of Treitz and transect the jejunum approximately 20 cm distal using a linear cutting stapler.

23. Bring the distal limb of jejunum through a window in the transverse mesocolon in a retrocolic fashion and juxtapose it to the esophagus, ensuring that it lies comfortably without excess tension or torsion.

24. Perform the Roux-en-Y reconstruction with approximately 60 cm of length between the esophagojejunostomy and the jejunojejunostomy to minimize esophageal reflux.

25. Multiple methods exist for creating the esophagojejunal anastomosis (Fig. 9.1):

    (a) A single layer running polydioxanone suture (3-0 PDS) using large, full-thickness bites is an acceptable approach. For this technique, a stabilizing suture is placed in the posterior aspect of the esophagus, with

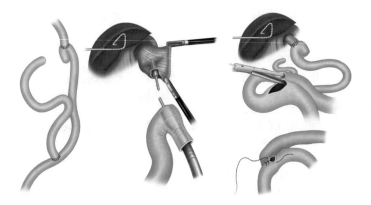

FIGURE 9.1 An EEA stapler can be used to create the esophagojejunostomy

the posterior aspect of the jejunum. The running suture is begun in the midline posteriorly, two over-and-over running sutures are then tied anteriorly.

(b) Alternatively, an end-to-end stapling device can be used, either with the entry point at the end of the jejunum or a more distal separate enterotomy in the jejunum.

26. Place a nasogastric tube across the anastomosis and ensure no anterior suture has caught the posterior wall.

27. Create the Roux-en-Y jejunojejunostomy 60 cm distal to the esophagojejunostomy (Fig. 9.1).

(a) If stapled: bring the two limbs of jejunum together using 3-0 silk sutures. Create enterotomies in each limb and introduce the stapler. Ensure adequate hemostasis of the staple line and close the common enterotomy with a linear stapler or with a two-layered suture closure.

(b) If sutured: perform a hand-sewn two layered end-to-side anastomosis using a running 3-0 Vicryl suture, followed by a row of interrupted silk sutures.

28. If a feeding jejunostomy is to be constructed: Place a purse string suture in the jejunum approximately 20 cm distal to the jejunojejunostomy.
29. Create an enterotomy in the center of the purse string suture and place the feeding tube through it.
30. Place 3-0 silk Lembert sutures to create a Witzel tunnel, effectively burying the jejunostomy tube. Create a stab incision to the left of the midline incision and bring the tube through it.
31. Suture the jejunum to the anterior abdominal wall using four-quadrant sutures with seromuscular bites through the jejunum. Tie these and ensure that the jejunum is fixed to the abdominal wall.
32. Place a closed suction drain in the area of the hiatus and esophagojejunostomy and bring this out through a separate stab incision.
33. Close the fascia using a running #1 PDS suture with 5 mm travel and 5 mm bites, the subcutaneous tissues using a 3-0 Vicryl suture, and close the skin using a running 4-0 Vicryl subcuticular suture

Chapter 10
Laparoscopic Roux-en-Y Gastric Bypass

Semeret T. Munie

Overview

- Ligament of Trietz identified, and jejunum is transected 50–70 cm distal
- Enteroenterostomy with biliopancreatic limb created
- Gastrohepatic ligament incised and left gastric artery preserved
- Gastric pouch created, and gastrojejunostomy created
- EGD to ensure no leak, and anastomosis is patent

Clinical Pearls

- Beware of internal hernias postoperatively (Fig. 10.1)

  - Most common site is Petersen's Space

- Antecolic anatomy prevents hernias and strictures
- Retrocolic anatomy is more physiologically normal

S. T. Munie (✉)
Division of Bariatric and Minimally Invasive Surgery, Medical College of Wisconsin, Milwaukee, WI, USA

© Springer Nature Switzerland AG 2020
E. Karamanos (ed.), *Common Surgeries Made Easy*,
https://doi.org/10.1007/978-3-030-41350-7_10

61

- Blind loop syndrome treat medically → if refractory re-ansastamose with shorter afferent limb

  - caused by poor motility and bacterial overgrowth

- Afferent loop syndrome → can balloon dilate or re-anastamose with shorter afferent limb

  - caused by mechanical obstruction of the afferent limb

- Efferent loop syndrome → can balloon dilate or find site of obstruction and relieve it
- Marginal ulcers will form on jejunal side of anastomosis

  - Lack brunner's glands and thus no HCO3 secretion
  - Treatment PPI, carafate
  - Rarely need to reverse, only in refractory cases

Patient Preparation

Supine with arms extended.

The surgeon stands on the patient's right side and the assistant on the patient's left.

Sequential compression stockings are placed prior to the induction of anesthesia.

Preoperative antibiotic administered within 1 hour prior to incision.

Weight-based chemical DVT prophylaxis administered in pre-op area.

Anesthesia

General anesthesia.

A Transversus Abdominis Plane (TAP) block can be used to improve perioperative pain control.

Additional Considerations

There may be some variations in the port placement, patient positioning, and placement of the roux limb in an ante- or retrocolic position as well as ante- or retrogastric position. This section discusses one combination of arrangements.

Operative Steps

1. A Veress needle is used to enter the abdomen at Palmer's point in the left upper quadrant and the abdomen is insufflated to 15 mmHg. Using a 0-degree camera, a 5 mm optical trocar is placed under direct vision.
2. A 12 mm port is placed approximately 18 cm below the xiphoid and 3 cm to the left of the umbilicus.
3. The camera is switched to a 30-degree angled 10 mm camera and placed through the 12 mm port. An additional 5 mm port is placed at the right midclavicular location slightly below the costal margin and a 12 mm port is placed in the right mid-epigastric region a palm's width medial and inferior from the right flank port.
4. A subxiphoid Nathanson liver retractor is used to lift the liver off the anterior stomach.
5. The transverse colon is lifted superiorly and the ligament of Treitz is identified. A jejunal loop is measured 50–70 cm distally. The small bowel is transected using an endoscopic linear stapler.
6. The mesentery is then divided using an ultrasonic device to the base. The distal end of the transected bowel is then measured 100–150 cm distally. This bowel is anastomosed with the biliopancreatic end of the previously transected bowel using a linear stapler to form the common channel. The common enterotomy is closed with a running absorbable suture.

7. Attention is shifted to the construction of the gastric pouch. The patient is placed in a reverse Trendelenburg position. The angle of His is identified and the fat pad at the esophagogastric junction is dissected off to allow visualization of the left crus of the diaphragm.

8. The lesser sac is entered by dividing the hepatogastric ligament at the level of the crow's foot. An endoscopic stapler is inserted through the created opening and first stapler is fired across horizontally, making sure the left gastric artery is preserved to provide blood supply to the gastric pouch.

9. A 32–36 Fr bougie is inserted and used to size the pouch with subsequent firing of staplers sequentially curved towards the left crus of the diaphragm.

10. The orogastric tube is pulled back into the esophagus. The previously transected end of the small bowel is brought up in an antecolic and antigastric position. Transecting the greater omentum may be required to allow the bowel to reach the gastric pouch.

11. A gastrotomy and enterotomy are made using ultrasonic device.

12. A gastrojejunostomy anastomosis is made by first placing a posterior running Lembert suture of the posterior wall followed by a running absorbable full thickness suture, followed by a running Lembert suture of the anterior wall.

13. An EGD is performed to evaluate the anastomoses as well as perform leak test by submerging the GJ into irrigation fluid.

14. Some omental fat is patched across the GJ.

15. The 12 mm port site fascia is closed with a 0 Vicryl suture on a suture passer.

16. The skin incisions are closed with absorbable sutures and skin glue is applied (Fig. 10.2).

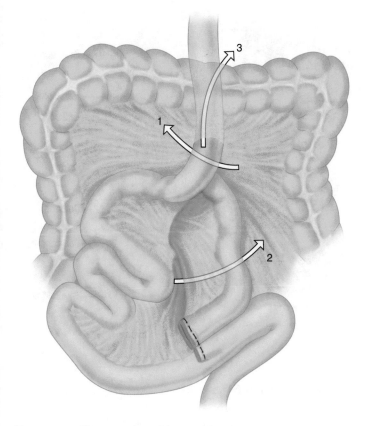

FIGURE 10.1 Common sites of internal hernias

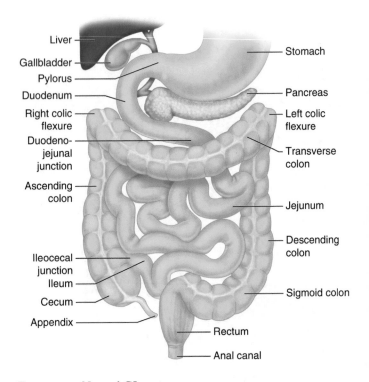

FIGURE 10.2 Normal GI anatomy

Chapter 11
Sleeve Gastrectomy

Semeret T. Munie

Overview

- Divide greater omentum off stomach, ligating short gastric arteries
- Size 36–40 bougie place, and pouch created by stapling from distal to proximal
- Leak test performed

Clinical Pearls

- Early tachycardia suggests anastomotic leak – always keep your suspicion for a leak low!
- Start with liquid diet, early satiety will be expected.

Patient Preparation

Supine with arms extended.

Sequential compression stockings are placed prior to induction of anesthesia.

S. T. Munie (✉)
Division of Bariatric and Minimally Invasive Surgery, Medical College of Wisconsin, Milwaukee, WI, USA

© Springer Nature Switzerland AG 2020
E. Karamanos (ed.), *Common Surgeries Made Easy*,
https://doi.org/10.1007/978-3-030-41350-7_11

67

A preoperative antibiotic is administered within 1 hour prior to incision.

Weight based chemical prophylaxis given in pre-op area.

Anesthesia

General anesthesia.

A Transversus Abdominis Plane (TAP) block can be used to improve perioperative pain control.

Additional Consideration

There may be some variations in the port placement as well as methods of sleeve sizing among surgeons. This chapter describes one arrangement.

The surgeon stands on the patient's right side and assistant on the patient's left.

Operative Steps

1. A Veress needle is used to enter the abdomen at the palmar point and abdomen is insufflated to 15 mmHg. Using a 0-degree camera, a 5 mm optical trocar is placed under direct vision at Palmer's point.
2. A 12 mm port is then placed 15 cm below the xiphoid and 3 cm to the left of the umbilicus.
3. The camera is switched to a 30-degree angled 10 mm scope and placed through the 12 mm port. An additional 5 mm port is placed at the right lateral flank slightly below the costal margin and a 12 mm port placed in the right mid-epigastric region a palm's width medial and inferior from the right flank port.
4. A subxiphoid Nathanson liver retractor is used to lift the liver off the anterior stomach.
5. The greater curve of the stomach is identified and an ultrasonic scalpel is used to enter the greater sac at the

mid greater curve by division of the greater omentum cranially with division of the short gastric blood vessels and caudally extending to a point of 4 cm proximal from pylorus. Any posterior gastric adhesions should be lysed.

6. A bougie (size of 36–40) is inserted through the mouth by the anesthesia team, advanced further and positioned at the lesser curve of the stomach.

7. An endoscopic linear stapler is used to staple lateral to the bougie beginning 4–6 cm from the pylorus and making sure not to narrow at the level of the incisura (Fig. 11.1).

8. Continue serial staples cranially up to the left crus of the diaphragm while staying next to the bougie.

9. The transected stomach is removed through the 12 mm port.

10. The sleeve staple line is tested for a leak with gentle insufflation while it is submerged under some irrigation fluid.

11. The 12 mm port site fascia is closed with an absorbable suture on a suture passer.

12. The skin incisions are closed with an absorbable suture and skin glue is applied.

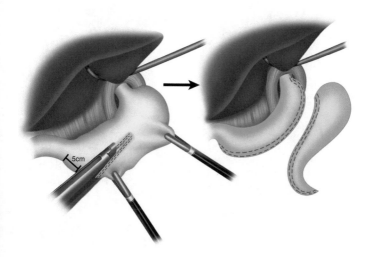

FIGURE 11.1 When performing a sleeve gastrectomy, it is really important to avoid narrowing at the level of the incisura

Part III
Small Bowel

Chapter 12
Loop Ileostomy-Laparoscopic

Shawn Webb

Overview

- Identify ileocolic junction, and measure 20 cm proximal
- Mark proximal to distal to ensure no twisting when making ileostomy
- Elipse skin and dissect to anterior rectus sheath, incise with cross hatch
- Bluntly dissect throught rectus muscle to posterior sheath, and incise to enter peritoneum
- Ensure adequate opening and then pass ileum through opening
- Close abdomen, and then create ileostomy
- Brooke proximal portion of ileostomy

Clinical Pearls

- Optimal ileostomy marked while patient standing
- If patient is obese, can core out more subcutaneous fat, and create an end ileostomy

S. Webb (✉)
Division of Colon and Rectal Surgery,
Henry Ford Hospital/Wayne State University, Detroit, MI, USA
e-mail: Swebb1@hfhs.org

© Springer Nature Switzerland AG 2020
E. Karamanos (ed.), *Common Surgeries Made Easy*,
https://doi.org/10.1007/978-3-030-41350-7_12

73

  – Can incise mesentery to get more length for ileostomy
- If ileostomy to distal, length will be limited by retroperitoneal attachments from colon
- Red rubber catheter use is attending preference
- Brooke ileostomy to avoid caustic bile on skin
- Parasomal hernia treatments

  – Sugarbaker repair with biologic mesh
  – Primary repair will recur
  – Resite ostomy if recurs and unable to reverse

Preoperative Considerations

Ostomy nurse marking and education to reduce any ostomy related complications.

Patient Placement

Supine with left arm tucked. Strap over the thighs. Strap over the chest vs a sticky pad on the bed. Strap over the head with head rolls. A Foley for bladder decompression. Prep the abdomen from below the pubis to the sternum, as wide laterally as possible on both sides. A laparoscopic drape with a wide aperture to allow wide access for triangulation.

Anesthesia

General.

Port Placement

Ideal port placement can vary. Three 5 mm ports will be sufficient. One port in left upper quadrant, one periumbilical, and one in the left lower quadrant staggered so is not in a direct line with the umbilical port when looking at the right lower quadrant internally.

Operative Steps

1. Scratch the skin where the previous stoma marking is located if marked by a preoperative ostomy nurse.
2. Gain access as above.
3. Place the ports as above, the camera port should be peri-umbilical with the other two as working ports.
4. Roll the patient with the left side down, a 15 degree rotation should be adequate.
5. Perform an adhesiolysis if it is pertinent.
6. Identify the ileocecal junction by the Veil of Treves (antimesenteric fat of terminal ileum).
7. Using atraumatic (Dorsey) graspers walk the terminal ileum up 20 cm from the ileocecal junction.
8. In order to maintain the orientation, lock the left upper quadrant grasper on the afferent (inflow) portion and the left lower quadrant grasper on the efferent (outflow direction). Assure there is no twisting of mesentery prior to locking the graspers.
9. Desufflate the abdomen.
10. Where the stoma is marked, ellipse a 2 cm area of skin.
11. If patient is obese, core out some of the fat.
12. Incise the fat in vertical fashion down to anterior fascia.
13. Incise the fascia anterior.
14. Bluntly dissect the rectus muscle with fat Kelly clamp.
15. Grasp and elevate the posterior sheath, can insufflate the abdomen at this point to help prevent grasping the bowel.
16. Incise the posterior sheath until you can fit two fingers to the second knuckle (approximately 4 cm).
17. Guide the bowel to the opening with the laparoscopic graspers.
18. Using a Babcock, grasp where the more cephalad grasper is (the inflow). Take caution to grab across the whole bowel loop before trying to lift it to avoid tearing the bowel.

19. Deliver the stoma and place a small ostomy rod between the mesentery and the serosa of the bowel loop. Secure the rod in place with a 3-0 nylon suture.
20. Can reinsufflate and evaluate for no twisting with direct visualization if concern for twisting.
21. Close port sites with a 4-0 Vicryl suture and dermabond.
22. Incise 2/3 of the circumference of the bowel at 1 cm away from the skin on the efferent (outflow, or caudal portion) with a cautery device.
23. Brooke the stoma first by taking the midline cephalad portion in full thickness fashion at its edge with a 4-0 Vicryl suture. Take a seromuscular bite 3-4 cm directly midline cephalad. Then take a dermal bite. Snap this without tying. Repeat the same step for the "3 o'clock" and "9 o'clock" position on the afferent portion. Tie these sutures with care to evert the mucosa and bud the stoma (Fig. 12.1).
24. The remaining stitches should all be interrupted securing the stoma to the skin circumferentially until all fat is covered. Usually 2 stitches between each "Brookeing stitch" and 3 stitches along the efferent loop will be sufficient.
25. Secure the ostomy appliance.
26. Can remove the foley at the end of the case.

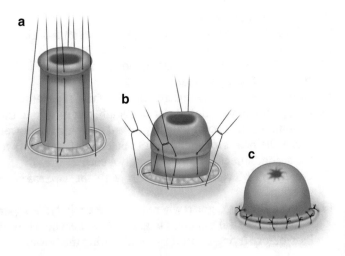

Figure 12.1 Brookeing of the ileostomy

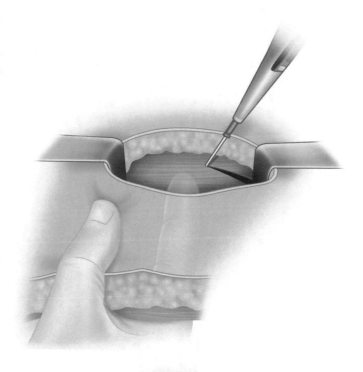

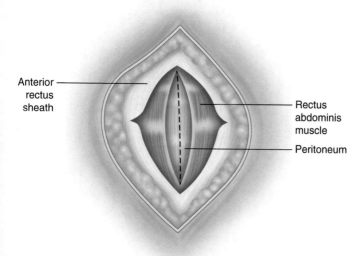

Anterior rectus sheath

Rectus abdominis muscle

Peritoneum

Chapter 13
Loop Ileostomy/ Colostomy Reversal

Shawn Webb

Overview

- Ellipse skin around ostomy and carry down to anterior rectus sheath
- Free ostomy from anterior and posterior rectus sheaths, and lyse any intra-abdominal adhesions
- Divide proximal and distal to ostomy, and then create anastomosis, irrigate abdomen
- Close fascia, and close skin over drain

Clinical Pearls

- Prior to reversal must get barium study, colonoscopy to assess for any distal strictures, and any masses
  - If patient has been diverted for prolonged period consider retention enemas to help alleviate postoperative diarrhea

S. Webb (✉)
Division of Colon and Rectal Surgery,
Henry Ford Hospital/Wayne State University, Detroit, MI, USA
e-mail: Swebb1@hfhs.org

© Springer Nature Switzerland AG 2020   79
E. Karamanos (ed.), *Common Surgeries Made Easy*,
https://doi.org/10.1007/978-3-030-41350-7_13

- When excising common enterostomy, ensure stapling across full thickness to avoid anastomotic leak, however, do not narrow anastomosis by taking too much tissue
- If unable to excise ostomy locally, convert to laparotomy
- Patient may have ileus postoperatively, advance diet after patient has bowel function
- There are multiple options for skin closure

  - Close primarily over a drain
  - Run purse-string deep dermal but leave skin open and pack with wet to dry gauze

Preoperative Considerations

Depending on the etiology of why the stoma was created, make sure the pathology that was diverted from is treated adequately prior to reversing the stoma. In discussion and consenting of the patient, make sure to explain the possibility of a laparotomy. The bowel prep for ileostomy can consist of clears for 24 hours only. For colostomy reversal, one should have a mechanical and antibiotic prep.

Patient Positioning

Supine with arms out. Prep wide enough that patient can be draped for a possible midline laparotomy if needed. Stoma does not need to be sutured shut, but can be if surgeon preferred.

Anesthesia

General

Operative Steps

1. Mark out an ellipse of skin either horizontal or vertical depending on the long axis of the stoma. If the stoma is taller than it is wide, a vertical ellipse will work best. The apices of the ellipse should be around 1 cm from the edge of the mucocutaneous interface. This allows the wound to close more easily.
2. Carry the incision through the dermis and fat in close proximity to the stoma down to the fascia. The fat should be able to be peeled away from the serosa of the bowel with a combination of blunt dissection with vascular providence Kelly clamp, cautery, and sharp dissection with Metzenbaum scissors where necessary.
3. Dissect the anterior fascia, rectus muscle and posterior fascia away from the stoma. If the aperture feels tight around the stoma, one can vertically incise the rectus sheath and the muscle to make room.
4. There will be subfascial adhesions on most cases that are important to lyse to get enough mobility of the ostomy.
5. Lyse the stoma loop free of itself so each loop is separate from the other.
6. Make a window in between the bowel and the mesentery where the bowel is healthy on both loops of the bowel.
7. Using a vascular providence Kelly, guide a GIA stapler through the window. GIA 55 will usually be adequate for the small bowel. GIA 75 is recommended for the colon.
8. Control the mesentery of the loop with vascular clamps and a 2-0 Vicryl suture ligature. Assure adequate hemostasis. Make sure when transecting the mesentery that the blood supply to the remaining bowel does not become compromised.
9. Cut the antimesenteric staple line corner of each loop of bowel off for approximately 8 mm. Dilate this opening with a vascular providence Kelly to assure in the lumen all the way and that the opening can accommodate one limb of the stapling device.

10. Insert one staple limb in each lumen of the bowel. Usually, the afferent (inflow) lumen is wider than the outflow lumen. Therefore, the blue side of the stapler should go in the inflow loop of bowel and the white side of the stapler should go in the outflow lumen.

11. As you line up and engage the stapler, guide the mesenteries away from each other to make the anastomosis antimesenteric. One way to do this is to put two fingers behind the bowel where you can't see when doing the anastomosis and spread the two fingers apart.

    (a) For a colostomy reversal, line up along the tenia choosing a tension free alignment. Sometimes you will have to spend time removing the epiploic appendages to free the tenia.

12. Remove the stapler after firing and evaluate the staple lines for hemostasis. If hemorrhage is noted, this is easily controlled with a figure of eight ligature with a 4-0 Vicryl suture right through the luminal aspect of the staple line.

13. Utilizing 6 Allis clamps, reappose the edges of the common enterotomy with care taken to grab full thickness of the bowel. In addition, one should offset the staple lines to avoid overlapping ischemic edges.

14. Once aligned, use a TX stapler (either 60 or 90 depending on the size of the enterotomy/colotomy) to staple across the enterotomy. Then use scissors to excise the extra tissue from the TX stapler (Fig. 13.1).

15. Utilize a 4-0 Vicryl suture in a figure of eight fashion for hemostasis. The stitches should go right through the staple line; do NOT imbricate the staple line for risk of staple line dehiscence.

16. Use a 4-0 Vicryl simple stitch at apex of staple line (some call it a crotch stitch or unzipping stitch.

17. Dunk the anastomosis back into the abdomen.

18. Irrigate as necessary. Cover the anastomosis with omentum if possible.

19. Close the fascia with an interrupted 0 sized suture in a figure of eight fashion based on surgeon preference. I use a 0 PDS suture on a CT-2 needle.
20. If significant contamination is present, leave the skin open to heal by secondary intention. If not, place a thyroid drain sized penrose in the base of the wound with the center of the drain in the center of the wound and both ends extending out of the apices of the wounds. Reapproximate the skin over the penrose without stapling the penrose to the skin. Then create a loop by stapling the penrose to itself over the skin staples.
21. Patient can have clears after ensuring that he is awake enough from anesthesia and advance as tolerated.
22. Remove the penrose drain in 3 days and the staples in 2 weeks if there are no signs of infection. If an infection develops, then remove the staples at this time.

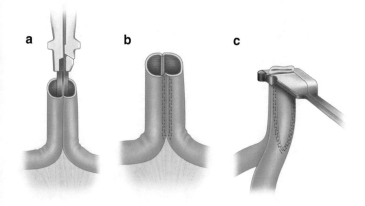

FIGURE 13.1 Stapled side to side, functional end to end ileostomy take down

Chapter 14
Stricturoplasty

Shawn Webb

Overview

- Perform laparotomy and adhesiolysis
- Identify stricture(s)
- Perform Heineke-Mikulicz, Finney/Jaboulay, or side-to-side isoperistaltic strictureplasty

    - Heineke-Mikulicz

        - Make enterotomy on antimesenteric border of stricture extending to healthy bowel
        - Close transversely in two layers

    - Finney

        - Make enterotomy between mesenteric and antimesenteric border of stricture extending proximally and distally
        - Strictured loop folded over itself to create a U shape
        - Opposed edges sutured together to create short side-to-side isoperistaltic enteroenterostomy in two layers

S. Webb (✉)
Division of Colon and Rectal Surgery,
Henry Ford Hospital/Wayne State University, Detroit, MI, USA
e-mail: Swebb1@hfhs.org

© Springer Nature Switzerland AG 2020   85
E. Karamanos (ed.), *Common Surgeries Made Easy*,
https://doi.org/10.1007/978-3-030-41350-7_14

– Jaboulay

• Make enterotomies between mesenteric and antimesenteric border of healthy bowel just proximal and distal to stricture
• Strictured loop foled over itself to create U shape
• Side-to-side enteroenterostomy created and closed in two layers

• Irrigate and close abdomen

Clinical Pearls

• Preop imaging used to assess number and location of strictures

  – MRE currently preferred study as it can distinguish between inflammatory and fibrotic srictures

    • Inflammatory strictures best treated medically

• Choice of strictureplasty (Fig. 14.1)

  – Short (≤7 cm): Heineke-Miculicz
  – Intermediate >7, ≤15 cm: Finney/Jaboulay
  – Multiple short strictures clustered: Side-to-side strictureplasty

• Improving preoperative nutrition is paramount; malnutrition will increase risk of anastomotic leak

  – Preop albumin should be >2

• Indications for strictureplasty

  – Diffuse strictures involving long segments of small bowel
  – Stricture in patients with short gut syndrome

• Always biopsy strictures left in situ to rule out malignancy

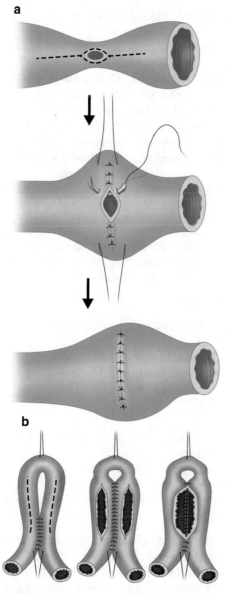

FIGURE 14.1 (**a**) Heineke - Mikulicz stricturoplasty, (**b**) Finney stricturoplasty

Preoperative Considerations

Patient selection is the most important factor when deciding to do a strictureplasty. Historically these were more common prior to the advent of better Crohn's immunosuppressive medications. Given the nature of tissue quality from a chronic fibrotic stricture of any origin, it is often better to perform a resection where feasible to get to good, healthy, pliable tissue. Strictureplasty is reserved now for patients where bowel conservation is a significant concern. It should be reserved for fibrotic disease that persist despite optimal medical management.

Current situations for consideration for strictureplasty are as follows:

- Multiple sections of small bowel involved diffusely.
- Stricture in patients who have undergone multiple previous bowel resections or long section removal (over 100 cm)
- Stricture in the setting of short gut syndrome

    Contraindications:

- Multiple strictures in a short segment (within 10 cm of each other)
- Active Crohn's disease in the segment
- Malnutrition (Albumin <2.0)

    Other considerations for operative planning include the length of the stricture segment

- <10 cm stricture is best served by Heineke-Mikulicz strictureplasty
- 10–20 cm stricture is best served by a Finney strictureplasty
- >20 cm strictures are best served by side-to-side isoperistaltic anastomosis

Prior to any operative intervention, some form of enhanced cross sectional imaging should be performed to evaluate the extent of the disease and the condition of the surrounding bowel. A CT enterography or a MR enterography should be done relatively recently to the timing of the operation.

The bowel prep can consist of only clears for 24 hours. If one is chronically obstructed, the patient may have been only on TPN.

Patient Positioning

Supine with arms out. All extremities padded well. Expect the operation to take several hours due to adhesiolysis. A foley should be placed. NGT decompression is recommended.

Anesthesia

General. Can consider a TAP block or an epidural for post-operative pain control.

Operative Steps

1. Midline laparotomy.
2. Lysis of adhesions meticulously. If there are dense adhesions and the preoperative imaging revealed an isolated section of disease to be repaired, you can limit lysis to area of focus. If there are multiple sections that need to be considered for strictureplasty, you should perform a full lysis of adhesions of the small bowel to assess the full length of the small bowel for diseased segments.
3. Locate the area or areas of disease.
4. Consider non-crushing bowel clamps above and below the area of the disease by 10 cm or so. This is especially useful in chronically dilated, obstructed bowel.
5. Assess which technique is to be used based on length of diseased bowel

   (a) Heineke-Mikulicz (<10 cm)

      • Incise the antimesenteric border full thickness into the lumen extending the incision 2 cm beyond the diseased segment into the healthy bowel.

- Evaluate the mucosa and biopsy it to rule out a malignancy if it appears concerning.
- Put two retraction sutures at the center of the stricture to pull the incision transversely to better align the suture line.
- Technique of closure can vary among surgeons. The goal is good apposition of mucosa to mucosa. This can be done with a running 4-0 Vicryl suture or interrupted simple 4-0 Vicryl sutures or a Gambi style stitch. I tend to use interrupted sutures for better distribution of the tension.
- Based on surgeon preference, one could consider a second imbricating suture line. You need to be cautious here to avoid narrowing the lumen.
- Some textbooks have recommended clipping of the retraction suture with a metal clip for future radiologic identification.

(a) Finney (between 10 and 20 cm)

- Incise the antimesenteric pathologic part full length including 2 cm on either side of health tissue.
- Biopsy anything of concern to rule out malignancy.
- Place a retraction stitch at center point of one side of the incision. By retracting this one side, it will form a U out of the incision with the apex being the retraction stitch. The part of the incision opposite of the retraction stitch will be adjacent to each other as the inside of the U. The line of the incision on the same side of the retraction stitch will form the outside of the U.
- Form a backwall with interrupted silk 3-0 sutures to approximate the serosa of the back wall, or inside of the U.
- Run a 4-0 Vicryl suture for the back wall running the entire length up to where the common enterotomy loops over to become the front wall.

- Close the front wall with a running Connell stitch until the entire enterotomy is closed.
- Imbricate the suture line with interrupted 3-0 silk sutures.
- Clip the retention suture for radiologic marking and identification.

(b) Isoperistaltic anastomosis (>20 cm)

- Place atraumatic bowel clamps on the healthy bowel above and below the stricture by 10–20 cm away to allow enough bowel length to work with.
- Incise the middle of the stricture transversely to create two separate ends of bowel.
- Move the proximal end over the distal end so they lie adjacent to each other in an isoperistaltic fashion. Overlap the full diseased area of one end with the healthy portion of the other end to avoid points of narrowing.
- Create a backwall of interrupted 3-0 silk sutures for the full length of the anastomosis.
- Open both sides longitudinally along the full length of the overlapping section.
- Evaluate the open bowel for any areas of suspicion for malignancy. Biopsy suspicious areas and send for frozen section. IF any malignancy comes back, you will have to perform a resection with lymph node harvest if it is safe.
- Barring any malignancy, run the full length of the enterotomy closed with a simple running on the common back wall and Connell stitch on the front wall.
- Close the front wall with Lembert style interrupted 3-0 silk sutures. Mark one on either end of the anastomosis with a hemoclip for future radiologic identification

Part IV
Colon

Chapter 15
Laparoscopic Right Hemicolectomy (Medial-to-Lateral Approach)

Sanjay Mohanty

Patient Positioning

The procedure is performed with the patient supine or in stirrups/lithotomy/split leg position, with both arms tucked; the latter has the advantage of allowing the surgeon to stand between the patient's legs, minimizing ergonomic issues related to the direction of the dissection and the camera angle.

The patient should be secured to the bed; depending on the institutional practice and/or surgeon preference, techniques to accomplish this include bean bags, non skid pads, shoulder braces, and silk tape.

A standard skin prep from the xiphoid superiorly to the pubis inferiorly and laterally to the anterior superior iliac spine.

Once the procedure is underway, the patient will be placed with the right side up and the head down (Trendelenburg position); occasionally, extremes of patient positioning are required to maximize visualization.

S. Mohanty (✉)
Division of Colon and Rectal Surgery, Barnes-Jewish Hospital,
St. Louis, MO, USA

© Springer Nature Switzerland AG 2020
E. Karamanos (ed.), *Common Surgeries Made Easy*,
https://doi.org/10.1007/978-3-030-41350-7_15

Anesthesia/Preparation

General endotracheal anesthesia

Appropriately timed (within 60 minutes of incision) intravenous antibiotics covering enteric organisms (e.g., cefoxitin, ciprofloxacin/metronidazole).

Depending on the patient's physiologic status and comorbidity burden, more invasive monitoring (e.g., arterial catheter) may be required.

Consider adjunctive pain strategies (preoperative administration of acetaminophen, gabapentin, NSAIDs, TAPP blocks, and epidural catheter placement).

A foley catheter is placed using sterile precautions.

Access and Port Placement

The abdominal access can be achieved based on surgeon's preference (open/Hassan technique, Veress needle, direct visualizing trocar).

Generally, there are no firm rules for port placement beyond those of triangulating based on pathology/right lower quadrant.

The camera port location should be at the apex of the pneumoperitoneum; most commonly, a 10-12 mm camera port is placed in the supraumbilical position, which will also function as the site of exteriorization and extraction of the specimen.

Additional 5mm working ports are placed (usually 2-3).

Two ports are generally placed in the left upper and lower quadrants, roughly a handbreadth apart. The lower port should be placed approximately 2 cm above and medial to the anterior superior iliac spine.

The third can be placed in a variable (suprapubic, left upper, or right lower quadrant) position, depending on the patient's anatomy and pathology.

The midline site will be extended and act as the exteriorization/extraction site.

Operative Steps

1. After positioning the patient right side up in steep Trendelenburg, the small bowel is retracted out of the right lower quadrant, and the greater omentum is placed in the upper abdomen, exposing the transverse colon. Optimal exposure should allow visualization of the right colon mesentery.

2. Atraumatic graspers and an energy, clipping, or stapling device (electrocautery, bipolar energy, ultrasonic scalpel) will be required for division of the major vessels.

3. Identify the ileocolic pedicle. This is typically done by using atraumatic graspers to elevate the ileocecal junction toward the right lower quadrant and anteriorly toward the abdominal wall, placing the mesentery under tension. The pedicle is identified as a "bow string" (Fig. 15.1).

4. The dissection begins by incising the peritoneum below the pedicle, in a direction parallel to the course of the ves-

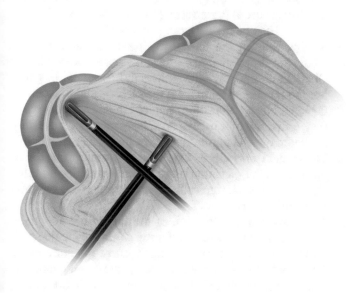

FIGURE 15.1 Identification of the ileocolic pedicle

sel. A wider incision makes this dissection easier. Using a blunt technique, the plane between the mesentery above and the retroperitoneum below is entered.

5. The duodenum should be identified and swept down. The dissection should proceed cephalad and laterally. The plane is largely avascular. Any retroperitoneal tissues are sometimes identified by a purple appearance; use this as a marker of tissues that should be swept down. Using your left hand to provide sufficient retraction and tension is key to making this dissection efficient, safe, and complete.

6. The ileocolic vessel is isolated and divided at its origin using an energy device, clips, or staples, ensuring the duodenum is safe from injury.

7. Next, identify the right branch of the middle colic artery. This is done by continuing the dissection as cephalad and lateral as possible, while always remaining aware of the location of the duodenum. The transverse colon mesentery should be elevated and placed under tension. The peritoneum is scored medial to the pedicle, and it is isolated at its base. After ensuring that the duodenum is safe, the vessel can be divided using energy, clips, or staples.

8. At this point, if the medial-to-lateral dissection is adequate, the only remaining attachments are located laterally. These are dividing relatively easily with good tension-counter tension from the surgeon and assistant.

9. Once mobilized, the colon is placed in its anatomic position. A division of the small bowel mesentery at the terminal ileum may be required to allow for a safe extraction.

10. The camera port site is extended, a wound protector is placed, and the specimen is exteriorized, ensuring that the colon remains anatomically oriented to prevent twisting of the mesentery.

11. After ensuring the location of the tumor and adequate margins, the small bowel and distal colon are divided and an anastomosis performed using the surgeon's preference. Commonly, a side-to-side, functional end-to-end ileocolic anastomosis using a GIA stapler, and a single fire of linear stapler is used to close the common enterotomy.

12. The viscera are returned to their anatomic locations and the fascial closure is performed in the typical fashion.

Chapter 16
Laparoscopic Left Hemicolectomy (Medial-to-Lateral Approach)

Sanjay Mohanty

Overview

- Sweep omentum over transverse colon onto liver
- Sweep small bowel out of LLQ
- Inferior mesenteric vessels identified, and dissection extended caudally and cranially
- Ureter and gonadal vessels identified and protected
- IMA isolated and divided (at its origin if high ligation needed)
- IMV isolated at inferior border of pancreas and divided
- Dissection of mesentery extended from splenic flexure to rectosigmoid junction
- Distal margin chosen and colon stapled
- Specimen exteriorized, and proximal margin then stapled across
- Colorectal anastomosis performed

S. Mohanty (✉)
Division of Colon and Rectal Surgery, Barnes-Jewish Hospital, St. Louis, MO, USA

© Springer Nature Switzerland AG 2020
E. Karamanos (ed.), *Common Surgeries Made Easy*,
https://doi.org/10.1007/978-3-030-41350-7_16

Clinical Pearls

- Rectum identified by splaying of tinea coli, and epiploica no longer present
- Sacral promontory is a reliable anatomic marker for identifying the IMA to begin dissection
- Performing medial to lateral dissection allows white line of Toldt to act as counter tension
- ERAS protocol

  - preop HSQ
  - preop entereg if opioid naive
  - TAP block
  - remove foley within 24 h
  - start patient on clear liquid diet and advance with return of bowel function
  - early, aggressive ambulation
  - preop NSAID
  - high carb drink 2 h before surgery

- Ureters cross medially at level of common iliac arteries
- Stents do not decrease rate of ureteral injury

  - Only help in identifying injury intraop

Patient Positioning

The procedure is performed with the patient in stirrups/lithotomy, with both arms tucked.

The patient should be secured to the bed; depending on institutional practice and/or surgeon preference, techniques to accomplish this include bean bags, nonskid pads, shoulder braces, and silk tape.

A standard skin prep from the xiphoid superiorly to the pubis inferiorly and laterally to the anterior superior iliac spine.

Once the procedure is underway, the patient will be placed with the left side up and head down (Trendelenburg position;) occasionally, extremes of patient positioning are required to maximize visualization.

Anesthesia/Preparation

General endotracheal anesthesia.

Appropriately timed (within 60 min of incision) intravenous antibiotics covering enteric organisms (e.g., cefoxitin, ciprofloxacin/metronidazole).

Depending on patient's physiologic status and comorbidity burden, more invasive monitoring (e.g., arterial catheter) may be required.

Consider adjunctive pain strategies (preoperative administration of acetaminophen, gabapentin, NSAIDs, TAPP blocks, and epidural catheter placement).

In the preoperative period, consider placement of ureteral catheter/stents.

A foley catheter is placed using sterile precautions.

Access and Port Placement

This procedure can be performed "straight" laparoscopically or with hand-assistance; the steps remain the same.

Abdominal access can be achieved based on the surgeon's preference (open/Hassan technique, closed technique/Veress needle, direct visualizing trocar).

Generally, there are no firm rules for port placement beyond those of triangulating based on pathology/left lower quadrant.

The camera port location should be at the apex of the pneumoperitoneum; most commonly, a 10–12 mm camera port is placed in a periumbilical location (either above or below the umbilicus).

Additional working ports generally number three, two of which are 5 mm, and one of which is a 12 mm port, to allow for passage of a stapler.

Two are generally placed in the right upper and lower quadrants about a handbreadth apart. The lower port should be placed roughly two centimeters medial to and above the anterior superior iliac spine. The lower port should be a 12 mm port if the distal division will be performed intracorporeally.

The third can be placed in a variable (suprapubic or left lower quadrant) position, depending on patient anatomy and pathology.

The specimen can be removed via a suprapubic extraction site.

Operative Steps

1. After positioning the patient left side up and in steep Trendelenburg, the small bowel is retracted out of the left lower quadrant, and the greater omentum is placed in the upper abdomen, exposing the transverse colon. Optimal exposure should allow visualization of the left colon mesentery.

2. Atraumatic graspers and an energy device (electrocautery, bipolar energy, ultrasonic) will be required, depending on surgeon preference.

3. Identify the inferior mesenteric vessels. This is done by elevating the rectosigmoid mesentery towards the left lower quadrant, placing it under tension. At the level of the sacral promontory, the peritoneum is incised from the origin of the inferior mesenteric artery to below the promontory, roughly 1–2 cm above the promontory. A wider incision makes this dissection easier (Fig. 16.1).

4. Once incised, blunt dissection is used to enter the areolar plane between the left/sigmoid colon mesentery above and the retroperitoneum below. This can be difficult early in the dissection, as the plane extends up and away from the camera's view. Identify the left ureter and gonadal vessels, ensuring that they are swept down with the retroperitoneum.

5. If this is for a cancer indication, a high ligation (close to the origin) of the inferior mesenteric artery is classically recommended. The peritoneum is scored along the base of the IMA origin to a point that is medial to the inferior mesenteric vein. A window is made in the mesentery, and the vessel is divided using an energy device, clips, or staples, ensuring that the left ureter is not injured and nerves present at the vessel's junction with the aorta are swept down.

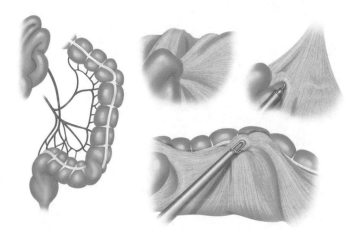

FIGURE 16.1 Left hemicolectomy

6. The dissection is continued laterally and cephalad to the inferior border of the pancreas, where the IMV is divided similarly using an energy device, clips, or staples, ensuring that the left ureter is not injured.

7. The medial to lateral dissection continues in a cephalad and caudad direction, from the splenic flexure to the rectosigmoid junction, which is identified by the coalescence of the taenia coli.

8. The rectum can be divided intracorporeally via the right lower quadrant port or in an open fashion through the suprapubic extraction site.

9. Once divided, the colon is exteriorized and resected. If a stapled end-to-end anastomosis is to be performed, the anvil for the stapler is placed in the proximal colotomy after the creation of a purse string. The proximal colon and returned to the abdomen and extraction site closed either temporarily or permanently.

10. The EEA stapler is introduced transanally and under direct vision, ensuring that the mesentery does not twist, the anastomosis is completed, and an air leak and/or an endoscopic assessment of the anastomosis is performed.

11. The viscera are returned to their anatomic locations and the fascial closure is performed in the typical fashion.

Chapter 17
Laparoscopic Low Anterior Resection

Sanjay Mohanty

Overview

- Inferior mesenteric vessels identified, and dissection extended caudally and cranially
- Ureter and gonadal vessels identified and protected
- IMA isolated and divided (at its origin if high ligation needed)
- IMV isolated at inferior border of pancreas and divided
- Splenic flexure mobilization
- Rectal dissection carried out, including the mesorectum posteriorly
- Distal margin chosen and colon stapled
- Specimen exteriorized, and proximal margin then stapled across
- Colorectal anastomosis performed

Clinical Pearls

- During preop workup, ensure either DRE, rigid proctoscope, or flex sig has identified distal extent of tumor

S. Mohanty (✉)
Division of Colon and Rectal Surgery, Barnes-Jewish Hospital,
St. Louis, MO, USA

© Springer Nature Switzerland AG 2020
E. Karamanos (ed.), *Common Surgeries Made Easy*,
https://doi.org/10.1007/978-3-030-41350-7_17

- Sacral promontory is a reliable anatomic marker for identifying the IMA to begin dissection
- When in "Holy Plane" during posterior dissection, pneumoperitoneum will help assist with dissection in this avascular plane
- Low Anterior Syndrome

  - Patients can have fecal urgency, frequency, clustered stool, and sensation of incomplete evacuation
  - Treatment varies, typically start with dietary fiber supplementation

- ERAS protocol

  - preop HSQ
  - preop entereg if opioid naive
  - TAP block
  - foley remains until POD 3 for pelvic dissection
  - start patient on clear liquid diet and advance with return of bowel function
  - early, aggressive ambulation
  - preop NSAID
  - high carb drink 2 h before surgery

- Ureters cross medially at level of common iliac arteries
- Stents do not decrease rate of ureteral injury

  - Only help in identifying injury intraop

Patient Positioning

The procedure is performed with the patient in modified lithotomy, with both arms tucked.

The patient should be secured to the bed; depending on institutional practice and/or surgeon preference, techniques to accomplish this include bean bags, nonskid pads, shoulder braces, and silk tape.

A standard skin prep from the xiphoid superiorly to the pubis inferiorly and laterally to the anterior superior iliac spine.

Once the procedure is underway, the patient will be placed with the left side up and in steep Trendelenburg position;

extremes of patient positioning are required to maximize visualization.

Anesthesia/Preparation

General endotracheal anesthesia.

Appropriately timed (within 60 min of incision) intravenous antibiotics covering enteric organisms (e.g., cefoxitin, ciprofloxacin/metronidazole).

Depending on patient's physiologic status and comorbidity burden, more invasive monitoring (e.g., arterial catheter) may be required.

Consider adjunctive pain strategies (preoperative administration of acetaminophen, gabapentin, NSAIDs, TAPP blocks, and epidural catheter placement).

In the preoperative period, consider placement of ureteral catheter/stents.

A foley catheter is placed using sterile precautions.

A rectal preparation can be used using saline and a tumoricidal solution such as povidone iodine.

Access and Port Placement

The abdominal access can be achieved based on the surgeon's preference (open/Hassan technique, closed technique/Veress needle, direct visualizing trocar).

The camera port location should be at the apex of the pneumoperitoneum; most commonly, a 10–12 mm camera port is placed in the supraumbilical position, which will also function as the site of exteriorization.

Three additional 5 mm working ports are placed.

Two are generally placed in the right upper and lower quadrants about a handbreadth apart. The lower port should be placed roughly two centimeters medial to and above the anterior superior iliac spine. The lower port should be a 12 mm port if the distal division will be performed intracorporeally.

The third can be placed in a variable (suprapubic or left lower quadrant) position, depending on patient anatomy and pathology.

The specimen can be removed via a suprapubic extraction site.

Operative Steps

1. After positioning the patient left side up and in steep Trendelenburg, the small bowel is retracted out of the left lower quadrant, and the greater omentum is placed in the upper abdomen, exposing the transverse colon. Optimal exposure should allow visualization of the left colon mesentery.
2. Atraumatic graspers and an energy device (electrocautery, bipolar energy, ultrasonic) will be required.
3. The mobilization of the left and sigmoid colon, splenic flexure, and the division of the inferior mesenteric vessels is carried out as described in the laparoscopic left hemicolectomy section.
4. The pelvic dissection may require a slight change in patient positioning, with less Trendelenburg. The dissection begins with elevation of the rectum and anterior retraction. The retrorectal space, characterized by filmy/areolar tissue is identified and developed sharply.
5. A sharp dissection (using electrocautery or energy device) is carried out along this "holy plane," which separates the presacral (below) and investing fascia of the mesorectum (above) (Fig. 17.1).
6. The hypogastric nerves, which descend into the pelvis and bifurcate into a wishbone configuration, should be identified, preserved, and swept laterally.
7. Anteriorly, be aware of the bladder, vagina, and, in men, the seminal vesicles/prostate.
8. Once the rectum has been mobilized circumferentially, ensure the level of transection and the tumor margin digitally and with an endoscopic examination, if necessary.

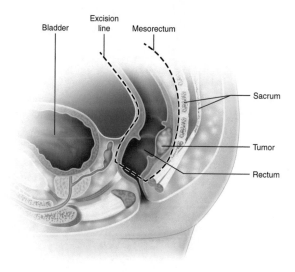

FIGURE 17.1 The 'holy plane' for total mesenteric excision during low anterior resection

9. The rectum can be divided with an endoscopic stapler intracorporeally or by using an open technique via the extraction site.

10. The rectum and distal colon are then exteriorized via a suprapubic incision with a wound protector in place. The colon is divided proximally and the specimen removed from the field.

11. An end-to-end stapled anastomosis is performed in the typical fashion, with the placement of the anvil into the proximal colotomy after placement of a purse-string suture and the introduction of the stapler transanally under direct vision. This can be done either via the suprapubic extraction site or laparoscopically after a temporary closure or use of an occlusive port (e.g., Gelport) of the extraction site. An air leak test and/or endoscopic assessment completed the anastomosis.

12. A diverting ileostomy can be created selectively.

13. The viscera are returned to their anatomic locations and the fascial closure is performed in the typical fashion.

Chapter 18
Abdominoperineal Resection

Sanjay Mohanty

Overview

- Mobilization of left colon from sigmoid to splenic flexure
- Inferior mesenteric vessels identified and ligated
- Proximal margin chosen and stapled
- Rectal dissection taken down to pelvic floor
- Perineal dissection from anus proximal to rectum
- Specimen removed, end colostomy created, perineal incision closed

Clinical Pearls

- Perineal dissection can be done in lithotomy or prone

    - Prone facilitates anterior dissection, but requires abdominal closure and maturing ostomy first

- ERAS protocol

    - preop HSQ
    - preop entereg if opioid naive
    - TAP block vs. epidural (attending dependent)

S. Mohanty (✉)
Division of Colon and Rectal Surgery, Barnes-Jewish Hospital, St. Louis, MO, USA

© Springer Nature Switzerland AG 2020
E. Karamanos (ed.), *Common Surgeries Made Easy*,
https://doi.org/10.1007/978-3-030-41350-7_18

- foley remains until POD 3 for pelvic dissection
- start patient on clear liquid diet and advance with return of bowel function
- early, aggressive ambulation

    if flap needed for closure, activity may be limited

- preop NSAID
- high carb drink 2 h before surgery

- Close perineal incision primarily in multiple layers, if due to bulky tumor or significant radiation changes, may need flap reconstruction (VRAM v Gracilis)
- Be wary of SBO after APR as small bowel can shift down into pelvis creating obstruction
- JP drain left in pelvis to facilitate healing of challenging perineal wound

    - Timing of removal is attending dependent

- Ureters cross medially at level of common iliac arteries
- Stents only help in identifying an injury, not in preventing one

Patient Positioning

The procedure is performed with the patient in lithotomy. The perineal phase of the operation can be performed either in lithotomy or prone. The latter requires closure of the abdomen and maturation of the end colostomy, but may facilitate anterior dissection and better visualization.

A standard skin prep from the xiphoid superiorly to the pubis inferiorly and laterally to the anterior superior iliac spine.

Once the procedure is underway, the patient will be placed with the left side up and in steep Trendelenburg position; extremes of patient positioning may be required to maximize visualization.

Anesthesia/Preparation

General endotracheal anesthesia.

Appropriately timed (within 60 min of incision) intravenous antibiotics covering enteric organisms (e.g., cefoxitin, ciprofloxacin/metronidazole).

Depending on patient's physiologic status and comorbidity burden, more invasive monitoring (e.g., arterial catheter) may be required.

Consider adjunctive pain strategies (preoperative administration of acetaminophen, gabapentin, NSAIDs, TAPP blocks, and epidural catheter placement).

In the preoperative period, consider placement of ureteral catheter/stents.

A foley catheter is placed using sterile precautions.

A rectal preparation can be used using saline and a tumoricidal solution such as povidone iodine.

Preoperative marking for optimal placement of the end colostomy.

If being done for cancer, depending on tumor size and involvement, multidisciplinary involvement (urology, gynecology, plastic surgery) may be necessary both for resection and for pelvic floor and soft tissue reconstruction.

Operative Steps

1. Access is achieved via a lower midline laparotomy.
2. A fixed retractor is placed, and the small bowel is retracted out of the pelvis and left lower quadrant into the upper abdomen.

   The mobilization of the sigmoid colon and, on occasion depending on patient anatomy, the left colon may be considered to facilitate colostomy creation. Generally, a mobilization of the left colon/splenic flexure is not required.

3. The lateral attachments of the colon are divided along the peritoneal reflection or "white line of Toldt." The plane between the mesocolon and retroperitoneum is entered and carried cephalad. The left ureter is identified, protected, and swept laterally.

4. Once mobilized to the midline, the inferior mesenteric artery is identified at its origin, and the vein at the inferior border of the pancreas, and divided. Care should be taken to clear any nerves from the IMA origin prior to division.

5. The proximal colon is typically divided at the junction of the descending and sigmoid colon. Once divided, the proximal colon is retracted carefully into the left upper quadrant and attention is turned to the pelvis.

6. The mesentery of the sigmoid colon is divided using an energy device or between clamps/suture ligature down to the pelvis and the pelvic portion of the operation is started.

7. The pelvic dissection begins posterior to the IMA entering the retrorectal plane until the "holy plane" is identified, characterized by areolar tissue, between the presacral fascia below (posterior) and the investing fascia of the mesorectum above (anterior).

8. The rectum is mobilized sharply circumferentially down to the pelvic floor. Distally, to prevent "coning in" (and reducing the risk of a positive circumferential resection margin), a cylindrical or extralevator APR should be considered, as the mesorectum of the distal rectum is absent. The dissection should be taken down to the pelvic floor, and liberal use of the digital exam will help in determining the level of dissection, particularly in patients with difficult anatomy. The anterior dissection, particularly in men, is the most difficult portion of the operation, and attention should be paid to avoid injury to the seminal vesicles. Retraction of

the rectum is maintained bu gently pulling the rectum out of the pelvis (cephalad), and using a narrow, ideally lighted, pelvic retractor.

9. At this point, a gauze sponge is tucked behind the rectum, and a decision should be made as to whether the perineal portion will be performed in lithotomy or in the prone position. Performing the procedure in lithotomy has the advantage of approaching the distal rectum from two places, which is helpful in difficult cases. However, it can also be difficult to visualize the anatomy appropriately when operating in lithotomy. Performing the dissection in the prone position mandates closure of the laparotomy and creation of the end colostomy prior to repositioning.

10. The perineal dissection begins with closure of the anus. A wide elliptical incision encompassing the sphincter complex is made and dissection proceeds into the ischiorectal space using electrocautery. The use of a sharp retractor (e.g., Lonestar) will greatly facilitate this dissection. Anteriorly, be mindful of the vagina in women or membranous urethra in men. A headlight can be helpful during this portion of the operation (Fig. 18.1).

11. The orientation should be reestablished frequently with palpation of the coccyx and insurance that dissection is proceeding anterior to this, until the perineal dissection meets the gauze sponge and the anterior/abdominal dissection.

12. The pelvic floor is divided, and the specimen is removed from the perineal incision.

13. The perineum is then irrigated, hemostasis assured, and it is carefully closed in layers.

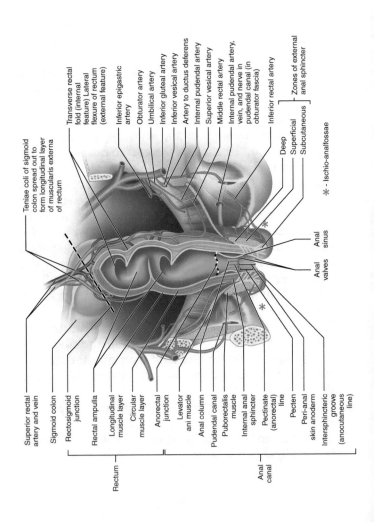

Chapter 19
Total Abdominal Colectomy

Sanjay Mohanty

Overview

- Mobilize ascending colon lateral to medial
- Take down hepatic flexure
- Dissect transverse colon mesentery off colon

  - if performing omentectomy, take gastrocolic ligament down keeping gastroepiploic vessels intact with stomach

- Take down splenic flexure
- Mobilize descending and sigmoid colon lateral to medial distally to rectum
- Transect proximally at terminal ileum, and distally at rectosigmoid junction
- Perform ileorectal anastomosis or create end ileostomy

Clinical Pearls

- Be wary of injury to duodenum or SMV
- Rectum identified by splaying of tinea coli, and epiploica no longer present

S. Mohanty (✉)
Division of Colon and Rectal Surgery, Barnes-Jewish Hospital,
St. Louis, MO, USA

© Springer Nature Switzerland AG 2020
E. Karamanos (ed.), *Common Surgeries Made Easy*,
https://doi.org/10.1007/978-3-030-41350-7_19

- ERAS protocol
  - preop HSQ
  - preop entereg if opioid naive
  - TAP block vs. epidural (attending dependent)
  - foley remains until POD 3 for pelvic dissection
  - start patient on clear liquid diet and advance with return of bowel function
  - early, aggressive ambulation
  - preop NSAID
  - high carb drink 2 h before surgery
- Ureters cross medially at level of common iliac arteries
- Stents only help in identifying an injury, not in preventing one

Patient Positioning

The procedure is performed with the patient in modified lithotomy.

A standard skin prep from the xiphoid superiorly to the pubis inferiorly and laterally to the anterior superior iliac spine.

Anesthesia/Preparation

General endotracheal anesthesia.

Appropriately timed (within 60 min of incision) intravenous antibiotics covering enteric organisms (e.g., cefoxitin, ciprofloxacin/metronidazole).

Depending on patient's physiologic status and comorbidity burden, more invasive monitoring (e.g., arterial catheter) may be required.

Consider adjunctive pain strategies (preoperative administration of acetaminophen, gabapentin, NSAIDs, TAPP blocks, and epidural catheter placement).

A foley catheter is placed using sterile precautions.

Preoperative marking for optimal placement of the end ileostomy.

Operative Steps

1. The access is achieved via a midline laparotomy.
2. The ascending colon and terminal ileum are mobilized by incising the lateral attachments along the fascial line of Toldt.
3. The right ureter and gonadal vessels should be protected and kept out of the dissection as you proceed cephalad toward the hepatic flexure. Be careful as you retract the ascending colon medially, as overzealousness can cause tearing of mesenteric veins and troublesome bleeding in the right upper quadrant.
4. As dissection is carried out onto the transverse colon, a decision must be made as to whether the greater omentum will be resected or left in situ. If resected, the lesser sac is entered the omentum is separated from the stomach, beyond or caudal to the gastroepiploic vessels. This is continued toward the splenic flexure, maintaining traction on the colon.
5. At the splenic flexure, be careful with retraction again to avoid inadvertent injury to the splenic capsule and troublesome bleeding in the left upper quadrant. If the visualization is difficult due to patient's anatomy or body habitus, attention can be shifted to the descending colon, where the dissection can begin and proceed proximally.
6. Once released, the dissection is continued along the descending and sigmoid colon, staying out of the retroperitoneum, identifying the left ureter/gonadal vessels. The dissection is sufficient once the rectosigmoid junction has been reached, identified by the coalescence of the taenia coli. At this point, the mobilization of the colon is complete.

7. The terminal ileum is divided with a GIA stapler. The mesentery of the colon can be divided with an energy device or between clamps and ties. If not being performed for a cancer indication, a high ligation of vasculature is not necessary and the mesentery can be divided close to the bowel wall.

8. The distal sigmoid/proximal rectum is divided at the level of the sacral promontory.

9. At this point, the operation can proceed to the creation and maturation of an end ileostomy or the creation of an ileorectal anastomosis, depending on the indication of the operation and the patient's status. In urgent or emergent scenarios, avoiding an anastomosis is advisable, with creation of an end ileostomy.

10. If performing an end ileostomy, the abdomen is irrigated. After verifying bowel health, adequate blood supply and reach without tension to the abdominal wall a disc of skin is excised measuring roughly 2 cm in diameter. A gauze sponge should be placed in the abdomen below the planned stoma site and the incision should be deepened carefully to the anterior fascia, which is then incised vertically.

11. The rectus muscle fibers are bluntly separated and the posterior sheath is incised vertically. The aperture should allow the passage of two fingers, and the small bowel should be exteriorized 5–6 cm, ensuring that the mesentery is anatomically oriented and not twisted.

12. All of the remaining abdominal wounds are closed.

13. The stoma is matured by excising the staple line and multiple interrupted sutures are taken, first with full thickness bites, then seromuscular bites superiorly and inferolaterally/inferomedially (approximating the shape of an inverted 'Y'), and finally, dermal bites. No seromuscular bites are taken at the mesenteric border to avoid compro-

mising blood flow. These are tied down and the stoma is everted. Additional interrupted sutures are placed full thickness and dermal around the stoma to ensure muco-cutaneous approximation. Ideally, the stoma should protrude 2–3 cm above the level of the skin.

14. A stoma appliance is placed (Fig. 19.1).

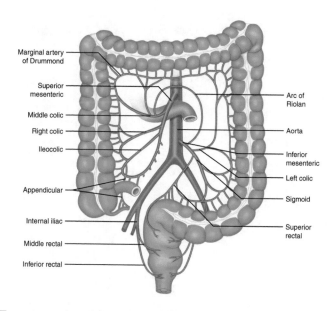

FIGURE 19.1 Arterial anatomy of the colon

Chapter 20
Open Partial Colectomy with End Ileostomy and Distal Stump Creation – Hartmann's Procedure

Ryan Shelden

Overview

- Mobilize descending and sigmoid colon by taking down white line of Toldt to the rectum
- Choose rectal margin and divide, place nonabsorbable stitch on rectal stump
- Dissect colonic mesentery with either energy device or suture ligation
- Choose proximal margin and divide
- Mature ostomy

Clinical Pearls

- Hinchey classification
  - I

R. Shelden (✉)
Division of Acute Care Surgery and Critical Care, Henry Ford Hospital/Wayne State University, Detroit, MI, USA

© Springer Nature Switzerland AG 2020
E. Karamanos (ed.), *Common Surgeries Made Easy*,
https://doi.org/10.1007/978-3-030-41350-7_20

123

  a: pericolonic phlegmon
  b: pericolonic abscess

- II: pelvic abscess
- III: purulent peritonitis
- IV: feculent peritonitis

- Rectum identified by splaying of tinea coli, and epiploica no longer present
- Proximal margin chosen at location that is not involved with disease

  - Diverticula may be present, but colon must appear healthy

- Ureters cross medially at level of common iliac arteries
- Stents only help in identifying an injury, not in preventing one
- Tagging rectal stump will help with identification on future reversal

Patient Placement

Lithotomy with bony prominence padding and both arms extended. A foley catheter is placed. The skin prep is with chloraprep. Depending on the indications of the procedure, an anorectal prep with betadine may be performed. The operating surgeon stands on the contralateral side of the anticipated colonic pathology.

Anesthesia

A general endotracheal anesthesia is required. A local anesthetic infiltration is preferable, but not necessary. A preoperative placement of epidural is encouraged but not necessary.

Landmarks and Skin Incision

The skin incision is typically midline, with vertical placement in relation to expected pathology. For example, a hypogastric midline incision is appropriate for a sigmoidectomy with cephalad extension of the incision around or through the umbilicus, if required.

The ostomy positioning is typically located within the triangle connecting the pubic symphysis, ASIS, and umbilicus. A preoperative review of the patient's mobility, belt location, and abdominal girth assist in the future stoma placement. Furthermore, a consultation with an enterostomal therapist regarding the ostomy location and the patient's mental preparation is invaluable.

Operative Steps

1. A 10–15 cm midline incision is created at the level of the anticipated colonic pathology with #10 blade. Hemostasis acquired using an electrocautery device, with the dissection continued to the abdominal wall fascia. Retraction of skin by a Weitlaner may assist in those with extensive adipose deposits.
2. A fascial incision is created with #10 blade followed by development of the preperitoneal space under the exposed midline fascia with digital dissection.
3. The fascial incision is extended along the length of the surgical site with the use of an electrocautery device.
4. The peritoneum is grasped with hemostats, lifted anteriorly, and sharply divided with Metzenbaum scissors thus gaining access to the abdominal cavity, followed by extension of this opening with cautery along the entire length of the surgical site.

5. Aerobic and anaerobic cultures acquired with a generous evacuation of the peritoneal fluid and debris with suction, if contamination is present.

6. A Richardson, Balfour, or Bookwalter retractor may be used for the exposure depending on the patient's habitus, the pathology location, and surgeon preference.

7. The colonic pathology is localized.

8. The colon is distracted medially and its lateral retroperitoneal attachment along the White Line of Toldt is incised with an electrocautery device. A blunt digital dissection allows for further development of this avascular plane. In the setting of an isolated perforation and/or colonic redundancy, the mobilization may be limited.

9. During the mobilization, the ureter is identified as it crosses the bifurcation of the iliac vessels.

10. A delineation between the diseased and healthy colon is made by a visual and manual inspection of the viscera. In the setting of diverticulitis, the resection only need to include the fibrous, boggy, or grossly indurated tissue with division through normal tissue.

11. Two mesenteric windows are created under the planned area of transection by scoring the peritoneum with an electrocautery device, approximately 1–2 cm away from the colomesenteric border.

12. A blunt dissection with hemostat allows the creation of an approximate 1 cm window.

13. A 75 mm blue load linear cutting GIA stapler is disassembled. The non-articulating handle is placed through the mesenteric window. The articular handle is then placed over the colon, ensuring an appropriate alignment of the two halves

14. After closing the stapler, the edema is allowed to egress out of the transection site by pausing 10–15 seconds prior to firing of the staple cartridge. Alternatively, non-crushing clamps may be used, followed by a sharp transection of the colon and placement of a 2-0 silk whip stitch of the non-specimen side.

15. The above procedure is repeated across the other mesenteric window flanking the colonic pathology.

16. In the absence of malignancy, a formal vascular-based mesenteric excision is not required. The mesenteric division may be performed with an energy sealing device or via a clamp-and-cut method as described below.

17. A mesenteric window is created approximately 4–5 cm away from the transected site as described above. A hemostat is introduced through the window and spread perpendicular to the axis of the intestine.

18. The arm of an additional opened clamp is inserted into the jaw of the first clamp to allow the second clamp to cross the mesenteric window. The first clamp is withdrawn and the second clamp slid down to the base of the mesenteric window, preferably with the angle of the clamp facing anteriorly.

19. The arm of the first clamp is inserted into the mesenteric window and slid to the apex of the mesenteric opening, followed by a clamp closure.

20. The mesentery between the two clamps is divided. A 2-0 silk suture is used to tie under the clamps, although tying on the specimen side clamp is not required. A 0 silk suture may be used if a larger vessel is appreciated within the clamped mesentery.

21. The above process is continued until the specimen is freed and allowed to be delivered out of the surgical field.

22. The mesentery and colon ends are observed for hemostasis. The use of sutures is preferable to the use of electrocautery in the regions of staples to prevent arcing.

23. A 0 prolene suture is placed through the distal stump to mark its location.

24. An ostomy site is selected in relation to preoperative considerations and anatomical restraints of proximal colon length. The location should pass through the rectus fascia (Fig. 20.1).

25. The skin in the planned site is grasped with a Kocher, lifted anteriorly, and then transected in a line parallel to the remaining abdominal skin to create a 2–3 cm circle. Hemostasis acquired with an electrocautery device.

26. A blunt dissection of the underlying adipose is performed with army-navy retractors until encountering the anterior

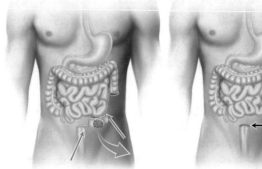

Rectosigmoid colon removed   Colostomy and closure of rectal stump

FIGURE 20.1 Hartmann's procedure

abdominal wall fascia. Alternatively, this fat may be excised with an electrocautery device if overly abundant.

27. A cruciate incision with an electrocautery device is created in the anterior rectus fascia followed by a muscle splitting technique to encounter the posterior fascia, which is bluntly incised.

28. The fascial opening should permit passage of two of the surgeon's fingers.

29. A Babcock is used to grasp the proximal colon stump and deliver it through the ostomy opening while preventing twisting. A wound protector may facilitate delivery. Upon exteriorization, the surgeon should be able to snuggly pass a single finger adjacent to the ostomy in to the abdominal cavity.

30. A minimum of 2 cm of colon (preferably up to 5 cm) should project above the surrounding abdominal wall skin. If the length of the proximal stump is insufficient, a further proximal division of the retroperitoneal attachments is performed.

31. Several optional interrupted seromuscular-fascial 2-0 Vicryl sutures may be placed.

32. An abdominal cavity lavage is performed.
33. A drain placement is typically unnecessary, but it remains surgeon dependent.
34. The abdominal fascia is closed per surgeon preference, such as continuous #1 PDS with bites taken 1 cm lateral from healthy fascial edge and advanced 1 cm from previous bite.
35. The subcutaneous tissue is irrigated and may be loosely closed or left open to heal by secondary intention. The site is covered.
36. The electrocautery device using the cut feature is used to excise the staple line of the proximal stump. Hemostasis ensured.
37. Interrupted tripartite 3-0 Vicryl sutures (incorporating dermis, full-thickness bowel wall at cut end, and seromuscular bowel just proximal to the level of skin) are placed in the 4 quadrants of the ostomy.
38. The four sutures are then tied causing the bowel to evert.
39. The remaining mucocutaneous border of the ostomy is developed with interrupted 4-0 Vicryl sutures incorporating dermis to the cut edge of the ostomy.
40. The abdomen is cleaned. The application of mastisol is advised around the stoma. The stoma appliance is tailored to fit, and applied.

Chapter 21
End Colostomy Takedown

Ryan Shelden

Overview

- Perform exploratory laparotomy and adhesiolysis
- Identify rectal stump and mobilize circumferentially
- Make ellipse around colostomy and dissect down to anterior fascia
- Free ostomy from anterior and posterior rectus sheaths and lyse any intra-abdominal adhesions
- Divide proximal to ostomy and ensure it reaches recutm tension free
- Create colorectal anastomosis

Clinical Pearls

- Tagging rectal stump will help with identification
- Prior to reversal must get contrast enema and colonoscopy to assess for any distal strictures and any masses

  - If patient has been diverted for prolonged period consider retention enemas to help alleviate postoperative diarrhea

R. Shelden (✉)
Division of Acute Care Surgery and Critical Care, Henry Ford Hospital/Wayne State University, Detroit, MI, USA

© Springer Nature Switzerland AG 2020   131
E. Karamanos (ed.), *Common Surgeries Made Easy*,
https://doi.org/10.1007/978-3-030-41350-7_21

- Ensure tension free anastomosis, as tension will increase risk of postoperative leak
  - If needed, take splenic flexure down to obtain more length
- There are multiple options for skin closure
  - Close primarily over a closed suction drain or penrose
  - Run purse-string deep dermal but leave skin open and pack with wet to dry gauze
- If at all concerned about the anastomosis, divert or revise

Patient Placement

The patient is placed in the lithotomy position with significant padding of bony prominences and both arms extended. A preoperative bowel prep is recommended, but remains controversial. A foley catheter is placed. A nasogastric tube may be considered. The ostomy is prepped initially with a betadine solution, the orifice whip stitched closed with a 2-0 prolene, and covered with a cellophane dressing such as ioban. The remaining abdomen is prepped with chloraprep. Betadine is used to prep the anus and perineum, along with instillation of a dilute 10% betadine enema. The surgeon stands on the patient's right side.

Anesthesia

A general endotracheal anesthesia is required. Preoperative epidural placement is recommended, if it is available. A skin infiltration with a local anesthetic is recommended but not required.

Landmarks and Skin Incision

The previous surgical site can typically be used for abdominal access, bearing in mind incisional hernias. The incision is made with a #10 blade and continued cephalad in to native tissue. An electrocautery device is used to continue the dissection to the anterior abdominal wall fascia. The fascia is sharply divided to allow passage of a digit into the preperitoneal space with further space development. The peritoneum is grasped with hemostats, lifted anteriorly, and then sharply divided to gain entry to the abdominal cavity. A lysis of adhesions is generally required to free the undersurface of the scar to allow extension of the celiotomy incision.

Operative Steps

1. Upon entry into the abdominal cavity, a generous lysis of adhesions is performed.
2. The distal colonic stump is identified. Only a limited mobilization is required.
3. The proximal colon is freed from the anterior abdominal wall.
4. The mucocutaneous border of the ostomy is divide. With hand retractors for assistance, the dissection is continued to the level of the anterior abdominal wall.
5. The fascial, muscular, and peritoneal attachments are divided to ultimately allow the ostomy to be introduced into the abdominal cavity.
6. The proximal colon is assessed for length and the ability to be seated adjacent to the rectal stump without tension.
7. Depending on the patient's anatomy and the surgeon's preferences, a variety of anastomotic configurations are possible. This discussion will review circular end-to-end stapled anastomosis (EEA).
8. On the proximal colon stump, a soft bowel clamp is placed approximately a palms breath from the end of the colon.
9. The end of the colon is sharply transected. A good blood supply is ensured and hemostasis is provided. The serosa is cleaned of fatty deposits for at least 1 cm proximal to the line of transection. The area of the anastomosis should also be free of diverticula.
10. A circumferential purse string suture using a 2-0 prolene suture or alternatively an autopurse string closure device is placed along the distal end.

11. An assistant will leave the surgical field to evaluate the perineum. A digital rectal exam is performed followed by serial dilation with graded dilators. The size of the largest dilator is then used to assist in selecting an EEA stapler size.
12. The selected EEA stapler is disassembled with anvil given to surgeon.
13. The anvil is introduced through the purse string suture into the proximal colon stump. The suture is then tied at the base of the anvil's post ensuring full closure around the post of the anvil.
14. The handle of the stapler is given to the assistant. The trocar is fully retracted and outer walls of the stapler lubricated.
15. With guidance from the surgeon, the assistant inserts the stapler through the anus and follows the curve of the sacrum to reach the apex of the rectal stump.
16. Upon appropriate placement by the assistant, the trocar is deployed adjacent to the previous rectal stump staple line.
17. The surgeon joins the post of the anvil to the trocar of the handle after ensuring no rotation of the either segment has inadvertently occurred. Successful union is denoted by a satisfactory click. Thereafter the two pieces should not be easily distracted from another.
18. The assistant turns the tension adjuster of the staple handle to approximate the handle and the anvil. Due to the variable height adjustment of EEA staplers, the assistance must monitor the degree of tension applied by observing the color-bar indicator on the handle. While closing, the surgeon prevents unwanted tissue (such as omentum or vagina) from entering the anastomotic region.

19. Prior to firing, a 15 seconds pause is instituted. The tension on the stapler is reconfirmed on the indicator. Some tightening may be required.
20. The safety of the stapler is released and the stapler is fired by squeezing the handles. Some pressure on the handles is held for a duration of 15 seconds and then released.
21. The stapler is removed and disassembled on the back table. Two complete rings of tissue should be apparent upon stapler disassembly.
22. A soft bowel clamp is placed at least a palms breath proximal to the anastomosis.
23. A rigid or flexible sigmoidoscopy is performed while the abdomen is lavaged to ensure hemostasis, patency, and absence of air leak.
24. Reinforcing the anastomosis with additional 3-0 silk sutures or silastic drain placement is not necessary, but remains surgeon dependent.
25. The fascia of the previous colostomy is approximated in accordance with surgeon preferences; for instance, with interrupted #1 PDS.
26. The abdominal fascia is closed per surgeon preference, such as continuous #1 PDS with bites taken 1 cm lateral from healthy fascial edge and advanced 1 cm from previous bite.
27. The midline skin is closed with either running subcuticular 4-0 monocryl sutures or closed with staples.
28. The colostomy site is closed over a penrose drain with staples.
29. The dressings are placed followed by application of an abdominal binder (Fig. 21.1).

Takedown of colostomy   **Side colon to end rectum coloproctostomy**

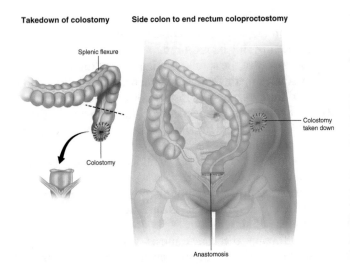

FIGURE 21.1 End colostomy reversal

Chapter 22
Laparoscopic Appendectomy

Hassan Nasser and Efstathios Karamanos

Overview

- Periumbilical port placed, followed by left lower quadrant port and supraumbilical port
- Patient placed in Trendelenburg position with right side up
- Omentum and small bowel swept into upper abdomen
- Appendix identified, window made through mesoappendix
- Appendiceal artery divided
- Appendix stapled off

Clinical Pearls

- Options for laparoscopic entry
    - Hasson entry
    - Veress needle
    - Optiview

H. Nasser
Department of General Surgery, Henry Ford Hospital/Wayne State University, Detroit, MI, USA

E. Karamanos (✉)
Plastic and Reconstructive Surgery, UT Health San Antonio, San Antonio, TX, USA

© Springer Nature Switzerland AG 2020
E. Karamanos (ed.), *Common Surgeries Made Easy*,
https://doi.org/10.1007/978-3-030-41350-7_22

- Can place right upper quadrant port instead of left lower quadrant port
  - Helpful in patients with retrocecal appendix
- If having difficulty finding appendix, trace tinea coli on ascending colon until they coalesce
- Ensure taking the appendix at its base as to avoid stump appendicitis
- Placement of 12 mm port is surgeon preference, as is use of energy device versus stapler to take artery
- Interval appendectomy can be an option in selected patients
  - Contraindication to interval appendectomy is presence of a fecalith

Patient Placement

Place patient supine.
  Left arm tucked.
  Foley catheter is placed to decompress the bladder.
  Prep abdomen with chlorhexidine.

Anesthesia

General anesthesia is required.

Landmarks and Skin Incisions

Umbilicus.
  Suprapubic.
  Left lower quadrant.

Operative Steps

1. Gain access to the abdomen using an open Hasson technique, Veress needle, or optical trocar at the umbilicus. A 5 mm or 12 mm port is placed.
2. The abdomen is insufflated with carbon dioxide.
3. A 5 mm 30-degree laparoscope is introduced through that port and the abdomen is inspected for any pathology.
4. A 5 mm suprapubic port is placed and either a 5 mm or 12 mm port is placed in the left lower quadrant (depending on the port placed at the umbilicus).
5. The patient is positioned in the Trendelenburg position with the right side up.
6. The cecum and appendix are identified.
7. The appendix is freed from any surrounding adhesions and the base of the appendix is identified. Sometimes the retroperitoneum needs to be divided. In cases of a retrocolic appendix, the white line of Toldt needs to be divided.
8. A window is created between the base of the appendix and the mesoappendix using a Maryland dissector.
9. The mesoappendix is divided using a laparoscopic harmonic scalpel. A laparoscopic linear cutting stapler with a vascular cartilage can also be used.
10. The appendix is ligated at the base using two pre tied Vicryl endoloops and then transected with the harmonic scalpel distal to the endoloops. A laparoscopic linear cutting stapler with a blue cartilage can also be used (Fig. 22.1).
11. The appendix is placed into an endoscopic specimen retrieval bag through the 12 mm port.
12. The base of the appendix is inspected to ensure hemostasis and evaluate the placement of the endoloops/staples.
13. Suction any blood clots or fluid from the surgical bed and pelvis. The authors' preference is not to irrigate the peritoneal cavity.

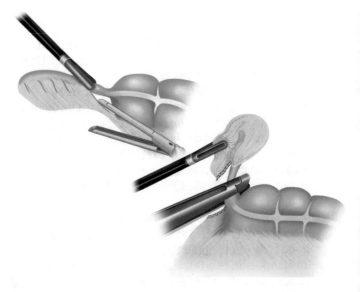

FIGURE 22.1 Stapling the mesoappendix and the appendix

14. Consider placing a drain if an abscess cavity is encountered.
15. The ports are removed under direct vision and the pneumoperitoneum is released.
16. Close the fascia at the 12 mm port site with a figure of eight 2-0 Vicryl suture. A UR needle is preferable.
17. Close the skin with interrupted deep dermal sutures using a 4-0 Vicryl suture.

Chapter 23
Open Appendectomy

Hassan Nasser and Efstathios Karamanos

Overview

- Incision carried down through fascia into abdomen
- Cecum grasped, and appendix exteriorized
- Window made through mesoappendix, and appendiceal artery suture ligated
- Appendix amputated

  - If sharply divided, burn mucosa with bovie

Clinical Pearls

- Choice of surgical incision depends on suspected location of the appendix based on point of maximum tenderness and imaging
- Ensure taking the appendix at its base as to avoid stump appendicitis

---

H. Nasser
Department of General Surgery, Henry Ford Hospital/Wayne State University, Detroit, MI, USA

E. Karamanos (✉)
Plastic and Reconstructive Surgery, UT Health San Antonio, San Antonio, TX, USA

© Springer Nature Switzerland AG 2020   141
E. Karamanos (ed.), *Common Surgeries Made Easy*,
https://doi.org/10.1007/978-3-030-41350-7_23

- Interval appendectomy can be an option in selected patients
  - Contraindication to interval appendectomy is presence of a fecalith

Patient Placement

Place the patient supine.
   Arms out.
   No Foley is required.
   Prep the abdomen with chlorhexidine.

Anesthesia

General anesthesia is required.

Incision

1. McBurney's point is identified (third the distance from the anterior superior iliac spine to the umbilicus). An oblique incision is made overlying that point. This is referred to as the McBurney's incision.
2. A horizontal incision can be made at the same point. This is known as Rocky-Davis incision.
3. A lower midline laparotomy can also be used.

The choice of surgical incision depends on the suspected location of the appendix based on point of maximum tenderness and imaging as well as suspected other pathologies such as Crohn's disease, peri-appendiceal abscess, or gynecological pathologies (Fig. 23.1).

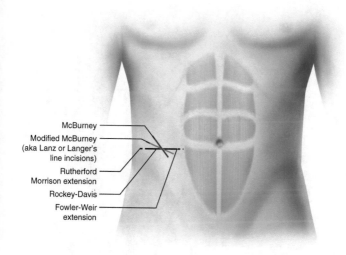

McBurney
Modified McBurney
(aka Lanz or Langer's
line incisions)
Rutherford
Morrison extension
Rockey-Davis
Fowler-Weir
extension

FIGURE 23.1 Other incisions in open appendectomy

Operative Steps

A right lower quadrant incision is made over the McBurney's point extending from the lateral edge of the rectus muscle to the right flank over the iliac crest.

1. The incision is carried down through the subcutaneous tissue, Scarpa's fascia, external oblique, internal oblique, and transversus abdominis parallel to their fibers (Fig. 23.2).
2. The peritoneum is identified and grasped between two forceps and then incised sharply using Metzenbaum scissors.
3. The abdomen is explored.
4. The peritoneal fluid can be sent for a Gram stain and culture.

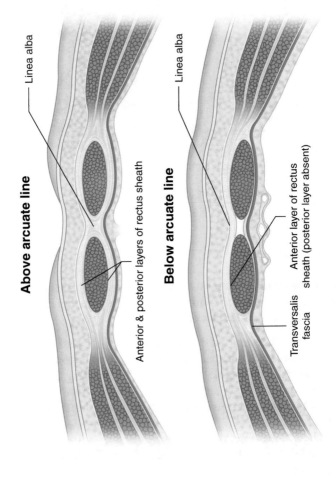

FIGURE 23.2 The anatomy of the anterior abdominal wall

5. The cecum is identified, grasped, and brought into the wound using a moist gauze.
6. The appendix is identified and exteriorized.
7. The cecum may need to be mobilized from its peritoneal attachments to allow a better access to the appendix, especially if retrocecal.
8. The mesoappendix is divided between clamps and ligated using 3-0 silk ties.
9. The appendiceal base is isolated using a right-angle clamp. The clamp is then moved 1 cm distal to that.
10. The appendix is then ligated.
11. A purse-string or a z-stitch is placed in the cecum at the base of the appendix using a 3-0 silk suture.
12. The appendix is then transected between the clamp and the ligature.
13. The appendix is invaginated into the cecum using a forceps and then the purse-string suture or z-stitch is tied.
14. The surgical bed is irrigated and suctioned and hemostasis ensured.
15. Part of the omentum is used to cover the cecum.
16. *If the appendix is not inflamed, the abdomen needs to be explored for another pathology.*
17. *If an abscess is encountered, an adequate drainage should be ensured, and a drain should be placed.*
18. The wound is closed in two running layers using a #1 PDS suture. The first layer includes the peritoneum, transversus abdominis, and internal oblique. The second layer includes the external oblique.
19. The Scarpa's fascia is then closed with an interrupted 3-0 Vicryl suture.
20. The skin is closed with staples. *Leave the skin open if there is significant contamination or an abscess is present.*

Part V
Liver

Chapter 24
Right Hepatectomy

Megan A. Coughlin and Michael Rizzari

Overview

- Take falciform ligament down
- Take right coronary and right triangular ligaments down
- Ligate short hepatic veins and identify and isolate right hepatic vein
- Perform cholecystectomy
- Identify right hepatic artery, ensure left hepatic artery patency, and ligate right hepatic artery
- Identify, isolate, and ligate right portal vein
- Transect liver parenchyma, ligating the right hepatic vein and then duct as they are encountered

Clinical Pearls

- Replaced right hepatic artery originates from SMA

M. A. Coughlin (✉)
Division of Pediatric Surgery, UT Health Science Center in Houston, Houston, TX, USA

M. Rizzari
Division of Transplant and Hepatobiliary Surgery, Henry Ford Hospital/Wayne State University, Detroit, MI, USA

© Springer Nature Switzerland AG 2020
E. Karamanos (ed.), *Common Surgeries Made Easy*,
https://doi.org/10.1007/978-3-030-41350-7_24

Right hepatectomy

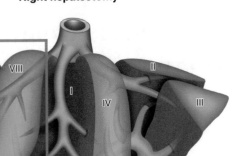

FIGURE 24.1 Segments included in a standard right hepatectomy include 5, 6, 7, and 8

- Replaced left hepatic artery originates from left gastric artery; will course through gastrohepatic ligament
- One liver, two lobes, four sectors, eight segments (Fig. 24.1)
    - Cantlies line runs from gallbladder bed towards the IVC, following the middle hepatic vein; this separates the right and left hepatic lobes
    - The hepatic vein system separates the liver vertically; the portal vein system separates the liver horizontally

Elevated central venous pressure prior to inflow/outflow ligation can lead to increased blood loss.

Patient Placement

Supine with reverse Trendelenburg.

Anesthesia

General anesthesia. Consider a preoperative transverse abdominis plane (TAP) block or an epidural for post-operative pain control.

Preoperative Preparation

Antibiotics.

Arterial and central venous catheter placement for monitoring and venous access.

Imaging available for review in the operating room.

Operative Steps

1. Right subcostal incision with midline extension to xiphoid or midline incision.
2. Inspection of tumor extension by palpation of the liver. Inspection of omentum, mesentery, small and large bowel and peritoneum for metastatic disease.
3. Take down the falciform ligament.
4. Intraoperative ultrasound of the liver to evaluate tumor size and relation to major portal and hepatic vein branches as well as middle hepatic vein anatomy and drainage.
5. Liver mobilization by dividing the right coronary and right triangular ligament.
6. Rotate the right hepatic lobe medially away from the diaphragm. Ligate the short hepatic veins communicating with the retrohepatic IVC. Divide the ligament over the inferior vena cava using a vascular stapler load if necessary, exposing the right hepatic vein. Pass an umbilical tape around the right hepatic vein.
7. Perform a cholecystectomy for clear exposure of the right liver hilum.
8. Identify the right hepatic artery, recognizing aberrant anatomy. Be aware of any small segment 4 branches, try to preserve these branches if they are coming from the right

hepatic artery. Check for the left hepatic artery pulse prior to ligating the right hepatic artery.

9. Expose the right portal vein branch, encircle the vein with a vessel loop. Occlude the inflow to identify the area of demarcation between the right and left hemiliver.

10. Ligate the right hepatic artery.

11. Ligate the right portal vein with a vascular stapler load. Alternatively, clamp and oversew the right portal vein with 4-0 prolene. Be aware of the small branch to segment 6.

12. Divide the inferior aspect of the caudate lobe to create a groove for the umbilical tape to "hang" the liver.

13. Follow the line of demarcation to mark the planned transection plane of the liver. Confirm the anatomy and resection margins with ultrasound.

14. Begin the transection of the liver utilizing an electrocautery device, ultrasonic dissection, crush and clamp dissection or hydrostatic dissection per preference. Obtain hemostasis and bile stasis by clipping or ligating small vessels and bile ducts. Vascular stapler loads may also be used to facilitate dissection of the liver parenchyma and to divide the larger portal and hepatic vein branches. The use of argon beam coagulation may be used to augment hemostasis at the liver edge.

15. Using a vascular stapler load, divide the right hepatic vein as you approach it in the posterior aspect of the liver transection; alternatively clamp and oversew the vein using a 4-0 monofilament suture.

16. As you approach the posterior liver hilum, use a surgical stapler to divide the right hepatic duct. Oversew the staple line of the right hepatic duct with a 5-0 PDS suture (optional).

17. Complete the transection and remove the specimen (Fig. 24.2).

18. Again confirm the inflow and outflow of the remnant left hemiliver.

19. Closure over closed suction drainage.

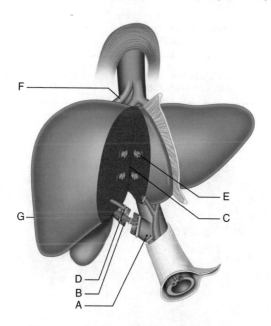

FIGURE 24.2 Structures to be divided with standard right hepatectomy: A. Divided right hepatic artery. B. Divided right portal vein. C. Cut edge of liver parenchyma. D. Divided right hepatic duct. E. Clipped branches along margin of transection. F. Right hepatic vein. G. Right liver to be removed

Extended right hepatectomy
or right trisectionectomy

Right hepatectomy
or right hemihepatectomy

Bisegmentectomy II + III
or left lateral sectionectomy

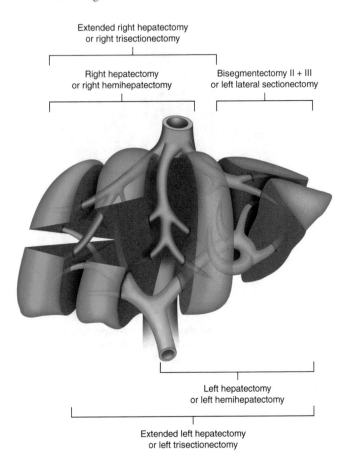

Left hepatectomy
or left hemihepatectomy

Extended left hepatectomy
or left trisectionectomy

Chapter 25
Left Hepatectomy

Megan A. Coughlin and Michael Rizzari

Overview

- Take falciform ligament down
- Take left triangular ligaments down
- Open gastrohepatic ligament and expose suprahepatic IVC, as well as middle and left hepatic veins
- Divide ligamentum venosum and expose retrohepatic IVC
- Identify and isolate left hepatic vein
- Perform cholecystectomy
- Identify and isolate left hepatic artery and left portal vein
- Ligate left portal vein followed by left hepatic artery
- Transect liver parenchyma, ligating the left hepatic vein and then duct as they are encountered

Clinical Pearls

- Replaced right hepatic artery originates from SMA

M. A. Coughlin (✉)
Division of Pediatric Surgery, UT Health Science Center in Houston, Houston, TX, USA

M. Rizzari
Division of Transplant and Hepatobiliary Surgery, Henry Ford Hospital/Wayne State University, Detroit, MI, USA

© Springer Nature Switzerland AG 2020   155
E. Karamanos (ed.), *Common Surgeries Made Easy*,
https://doi.org/10.1007/978-3-030-41350-7_25

- Replaced left hepatic artery originates from left gastric artery; will course through gastrohepatic ligament
- One liver, two lobes, four sectors, eight segments
  - Cantlies line runs from gallbladder bed towards the IVC, following the middle hepatic vein; this separates the right and left hepatic lobes
  - The hepatic vein system separates the liver vertically; the portal vein system separates the liver horizontally
- Elevated central venous pressure prior to inflow/outflow ligation can lead to increased blood loss

Patient Placement

Supine with reverse Trendelenburg.

Anesthesia

General anesthesia. Consider preoperative transverse abdominis plane (TAP) block or epidural for post-operative pain control.

Preoperative Preparation

Antibiotics.

Arterial and central venous catheter placement for monitoring and venous access.

Imaging available for review in the operating room.

Operative Steps

1. Upper midline incision.
2. Take down the falciform ligament.
3. Inspection of tumor extension by palpation of liver. Inspection of omentum, mesentery, small and large bowel and peritoneum for metastatic disease.

4. Intraoperative ultrasound of the liver to evaluate tumor size and relation to major portal and hepatic vein branches as well as middle hepatic vein anatomy and drainage.

5. Take down the left triangular ligament.

6. Incise the lesser omentum. Beware of replaced left hepatic artery.

7. Expose the suprahepatic IVC and the middle/left hepatic vein trunk.

8. Divide the ligamentum venosum and expose the retrohepatic IVC.

9. Pass an umbilical tape around the left hepatic vein. You may need to incise the liver to expose the branch point of the middle and left hepatic vein.

10. Perform cholecystectomy.

11. Lower the hilar plate, expose the left hepatic artery and left portal vein.

12. Expose left portal vein, encircle the vein with vessel loop. Occlude the inflow to identify the area of demarcation between right and left hemiliver.

13. Expose and be aware of aberrant anatomy of the left hepatic artery and divide. Be aware of segment 4 branches from the left hepatic artery and preserve if possible.

14. Ligate the left portal vein with a vascular stapler load. Alternatively, clamp and oversew with 4-0 prolene sutures. Be aware of small branches to segment 1.

15. Using ultrasound, mark the line of dissection of the left lobe with electrocautery, extending into the gallbladder fossa, noting the path and branches of the left hepatic vein.

16. Pass the umbilical tape posteriorly behind the liver and through the hilum to guide liver transection and "hang" the liver.

17. Begin transection of the liver utilizing electrocautery, ultrasonic dissection, crush and clamp dissection or hydrostatic dissection per preference. Obtain hemostasis and bile stasis by clipping or ligating small vessels and bile ducts. Vascular stapler loads may also be used to facilitate dissection of the liver parenchyma and to divide larger portal and hepatic vein branches. Argon beam coagulation may be used to augment hemostasis at the liver edge.

18. Using a vascular stapler load, divide the left hepatic vein as you approach it in the posterior aspect of the liver transection; alternatively clamp and oversew the vein using 4-0 prolene suture.
19. As you approach the posterior liver hilum, use a surgical stapler to divide the left hepatic duct. Oversew the staple line of the left hepatic duct with 5-0 PDS sutures (optional).
20. Complete the transection and remove the specimen (Fig. 25.1).
21. Again confirm inflow and outflow of the remnant right hemiliver.
22. Ensure adequate hemostasis and close over closed suction drainage.

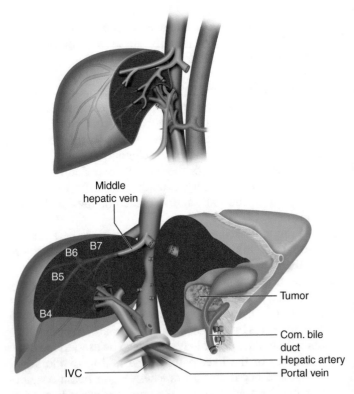

FIGURE 25.1 Left hepatectomy

Part VI
Pancreas

Chapter 26
Open Distal Pancreatectomy

Konstantinos Chouliaras and Mio Kitano

Overview

- Divide gastrocolic ligament to enter lesser sac
- If preserving spleen, dissect splenic artery and vein off superior border of pancreas
- If performing concomitant splenectomy, take splenocolic, gastrosplenic, splenophrenic, splenorenal ligaments down
- Determine transection point of pancreas, and divide pancreas
- Ligate splenic artery and vein if performing splenectomy

Clinical Pearls

- Gastrosplenic ligament is only splenic ligament that contains vasculature
- Dividing splenophrenic ligament allows spleen to remain retracted while dissection is carried out

K. Chouliaras (✉)
Department of Surgery, Wake Forest University,
Winston-Salem, NC, USA

M. Kitano
Division of Surgical Oncology and Endocrine Surgery, UT Health
San Antonio, San Antonio, TX, USA

© Springer Nature Switzerland AG 2020   161
E. Karamanos (ed.), *Common Surgeries Made Easy*,
https://doi.org/10.1007/978-3-030-41350-7_26

- If patient has chronic pancreatitis, avoid stapling across pancreas, and oversew to avoid pancreatic leaks
- JP drain placement is attending dependent

Patient Positioning

The patient is placed supine with both arms extended.

It is important to prep the skin to the level of the nipples.

Anesthesia

General endotracheal anesthesia is needed.

An epidural catheter or US-guided long-acting anesthetic blocks may be used to assist with pain control.

Vaccines against encapsulated bacteria should be administered if a concurrent splenectomy is to be performed. Patients should receive the vaccines on the day of discharge or 14 days post-op (whichever comes first).

A foley catheter is placed for close urine output measurement.

Operative Steps

1. An upper midline laparotomy or left subcostal incision is made.
2. The entire abdomen is explored and inspected for any evidence of metastatic disease. Close attention should be paid to examining and palpating the liver. Any suspicious lesions should be biopsied and sent for frozen section. If a frozen section shows evidence of metastasis, surgical resection should not be pursued.
3. A fixed retractor is placed (a Thompson retractor provides excellent exposure but a variety of other retractors can be used such as a Bookwalter, Omni-tract, Balfour etc.).
4. The lesser sac is entered after dividing the gastrocolic ligament, exposing the pancreas.

5. The lesion is palpated or assessed with the US intraopera-
tively to delineate the exact borders and confirm the location and resectability with the chosen procedure.

Spleen-Preserving Distal Pancreatectomy

1. The superior border of the pancreas is dissected proximal
to the lesion of interest to isolate the splenic artery and
the vein. For a spleen-preserving distal pancreatectomy,
small tributaries from the splenic artery and the vein need
to be meticulously ligated or clipped to completely free
the tail of the pancreas from the vascular bundle.
2. The inferior border of the pancreas is then dissected.
3. The plane of transection is confirmed and a tunnel is created. Two stay sutures can be placed at the superior and
inferior border of the pancreatic remnant to facilitate with
hemostasis (Fig. 26.1).

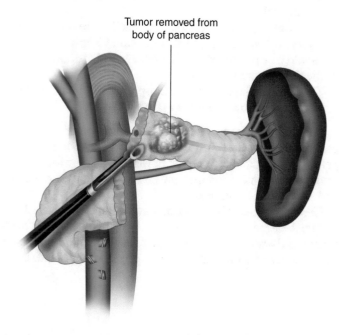

Tumor removed from
body of pancreas

FIGURE 26.1 Spleen preserving distal pancreatectomy

In Cases of Combined Splenectomy

1. It is often challenging to preserve the spleen due to intimate relationship of splenic artery and vein to the pancreatic parenchyma.
2. Additionally, the spleen should not be preserved in case of tumor involvement of the splenic vasculature or evidence of splenic vein thrombosis.
3. The splenophrenic, splenocolic, splenorenal, and gastrosplenic ligaments are divided.
4. The gastrosplenic and splenocolic ligaments contain the short gastric vessels and the left gastroepiploic vessels and careful hemostasis is obtained, usually with an advanced energy device (bipolar or ultrasonic dissector) or with suture ligature.
5. The spleen is fully mobilized and retracted medially.
6. The splenic vasculature is approached and isolated from the posterior aspect of the pancreas as spleen is medialized.
7. A vascular stapler load may be used to seal the splenic artery and vein or may be suture ligated. The splenic artery should be divided first to minimize blood loss and to drain the blood from the spleen.
8. The midline laparotomy is closed in a standard fashion. The chevron incision is closed in two layers.

For both a spleen-preserving and a non-preserving distal pancreatectomy, there are several ways to divide the pancreas parenchyma including stapling devices, division with an electrocautery device or scalpel and oversewing the parenchyma with full thickness sutures.

Careful hemostasis is obtained and wound is irrigated.

The decision to place a drain depends on the surgeon preference and also based on the texture of the pancreas, the size of the pancreatic duct and the type of pathology treated.

Chapter 27
Laparoscopic Distal Pancreatectomy

Konstantinos Chouliaras and Mio Kitano

Overview

- Divide gastrocolic ligament to enter lesser sac
- Dissect the inferior border of the pancreas
- Posterior tunnel created proximal to lesion; divide pancreas
- If preserving spleen, will need to dissect splenic tributaries with energy device or clips
- If performing concomitant splenectomy, staple across splenic artery and vein
- Dissect splenocolic, gastrosplenic, splenophrenic, splenorenal ligaments down

Clinical Pearls

- Avoid excessive traction on the splenic side to prevent capsular tears

K. Chouliaras (✉)
Department of Surgery, Wake Forest University,
Winston-Salem, NC, USA

M. Kitano
Division of Surgical Oncology and Endocrine Surgery, UT Health
San Antonio, San Antonio, TX, USA

© Springer Nature Switzerland AG 2020   165
E. Karamanos (ed.), *Common Surgeries Made Easy*,
https://doi.org/10.1007/978-3-030-41350-7_27

- Gastrosplenic ligament is only splenic ligament that contains vasculature
- Dividing splenophrenic ligament allows spleen to remain retracted while dissection is carried out
- If patient has chronic pancreatitis, use energy device and oversew to avoid pancreatic leaks
- JP drain placement is attending dependent

Patient Positioning

The patient is placed supine with both arms extended.

It is important to prep the skin to the level of the nipples.

The patient is secured well to the operative table and all the pressure points are padded (Fig. 27.1).

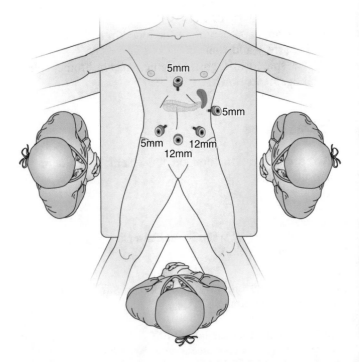

FIGURE 27.1 Surgeon's positioning during laparoscopic splenectomy

Anesthesia

General endotracheal anesthesia is needed.

Vaccines against encapsulated bacteria should be administered if a concurrent splenectomy is performed. The patients should receive the vaccines on the day of discharge or 14 days post-op (whichever comes first).

A foley catheter is placed for close urine output measurement.

Operative Steps

1. An open Hasson technique or a Veress needle technique may be utilized to establish the pneumoperitoneum. The Veress needle is placed in the left upper quadrant after ensuring adequate decompression of the stomach via an orogastric or nasogastric tube.
2. A diagnostic laparoscopy is performed to assess for peritoneal spread or possible liver involvement.
3. Three more ports are placed, one 5 mm to the RUQ and one 12 mm to the LUQ as well as one 5 mm to the left anterior axillary line. Of note, port selection may vary based on the body habitus or the surgeon's preference.
4. The patient is placed in reverse Trendelenburg to facilitate exposure.
5. The gastrocolic ligament is divided with the help of an advanced bipolar or ultrasonic energy device.
6. The splenic flexure may need to be mobilized to gain adequate exposure to the tail of the pancreas.
7. A fan retractor may be useful to provide better visualization of the pancreas and occasionally some attachments may have to be divided between the posterior surface of the stomach and the pancreas.
8. The pancreatic lesion is visualized and can be better assessed with intraoperative ultrasound to confirm the location of the lesion, area of transection, and resectability.
9. The inferior border of the pancreas is dissected.

Spleen-Preserving Distal Pancreatectomy

1. A tunnel is created proximal to the lesion of interest with caution as the splenic vessels lay posteriorly and may lead to troublesome bleeding.
2. A stapling device is used for the pancreatic transection. The stapler load may be covered/buttressed as it may decrease the risk of a leak.
3. The pancreas is then further dissected off of the retroperitoneum from medial to lateral.
4. Tributaries to the splenic vessels will have to be clipped or sealed with the energy device.
5. In cases with problematic bleeding, the splenic vessels may have to be doubly stapled, proximally and distally in order to achieve hemostasis, making sure that the short gastric vessels are preserved (Warshaw technique).
6. The specimen is placed in a retrieval bag.
7. A drain may be placed based on the surgeon's preference.
8. One of the ports is then extended in size to remove the specimen and is subsequently irrigated and closed in standard fashion.

If Splenectomy Is Also Performed

1. The splenic vessels are transected with the use of a vascular stapler load at the level of the pancreatic transection.
2. The short gastric vessels are divided and the avascular splenocolic and splenophrenic ligaments are divided with the help of an energy device.
3. All remaining attachments are divided. Typically there are only avascular retroperitoneal attachments remaining.

Chapter 28
Pancreaticoduodenectomy (Whipple Procedure)

Konstantinos Chouliaras and Mio Kitano

Overview

Its easiest to divide the whipple into 4 broad categories: exploration, dissection, division, reconstruction

- Exploration of the abdominal cavity to rule out gross metastatic disease
- Dissection

  - Open lesser sac by taking gastrocolic ligament down
  - Kocher maneuver
  - Cholecystectomy
  - Dissection of inferior pancreatic border, and identification of IMV traced proximally towards pancreas
  - Portal dissection
  - GDA identified, isolated, and ligated
      ensure hepatic artery patent prior to ligation
  - Retropancreatic tunnel dissected

K. Chouliaras (✉)
Department of Surgery, Wake Forest University,
Winston-Salem, NC, USA

M. Kitano
Division of Surgical Oncology and Endocrine Surgery, UT Health
San Antonio, San Antonio, TX, USA

© Springer Nature Switzerland AG 2020   169
E. Karamanos (ed.), *Common Surgeries Made Easy*,
https://doi.org/10.1007/978-3-030-41350-7_28

- Division

  - Distal stomach vs duodenum transected (attending dependent)
  - Proximal jejunum transected
  - Pancreatic parenchyma transected, and pancreas dissected off the SMA and PV

- Reconstruction

  - Pancreaticojejunostomy → duct to mucosa vs. invagination (attending dependent)
  - Choledocojejunostomy
  - Gastrojejunostomy

Clinical Pearls

- Delayed gastric emptying is the most common postoperative complication
- Full Kocher maneuver: Inferior to right renal vein, superior to portal vein, medial to pancreatic head
- GDA stump blowout mortality 50%

  - Will have sentinel bleed → IR for stent in hepatic artery across GDA

- Pancreatic Fistula occurs in 15–20% of patients

  - Type A: asymptomatic, but biochemically confirmed with drain amylase >3x serum, or drain output >400 mL/day
  - Type B: pancreatic fistula requiring an intervention: TPN, additional drain placement
  - Type C: anastomotic failure requiring operative intervention

- Contraindication to surgical resection

  - Tumor abutting CA or HA
  - Encasement of >180 degrees of SMA
  - Encasement of SMV with long segment of occlusion of SMV/PV

- Borderline Resectability
  - Venous distortion of SMV/PV
  - Short segment occlusion SMV/PV
  - Encasement of <180 degrees of SMA
  - Encasement of GDA up to HA
- Vascular reconstruction options of SMV
  - Internal Jugular, Femoral Vein, Greater Saphenous Vein, Renal Vein, Synthetic (PTFE), Cryovein

Patient Positioning

The patient is placed supine with both arms extended.

It is important to prep the skin to the level of the nipples.

It is important to prep the neck and/or the groin if portal vein resection is planned.

Anesthesia

General endotracheal anesthesia is needed.

An epidural catheter or a US-guided long-acting anesthetic blocks may be used to assist with pain control.

A foley catheter is placed for close urine output measurement.

Large bore IV access should be secured +/− arterial line for hemodynamic monitoring.

Operative Steps

1. A midline laparotomy incision is made from the xiphoid to below the umbilicus. Alternatively, a left subcostal incision is made.
2. The abdomen is explored for evidence of peritoneal disease. The liver is examined, particularly for evidence of metastatic disease. Any suspicious lesions are biopsied and sent for frozen section.

3. The falciform ligament is taken down with an electrocautery device and a fixed retractor is placed (Thompson retractor provides excellent exposure but a variety of other retractors can be used such as Bookwalter, Omni-tract, Balfour, etc.).

The operation can be divided into two main parts: resection and reconstruction.

Pancreatic Resection

1. An extensive Kocher maneuver is performed, mobilizing the duodenum, starting from lateral to medial. This is usually bloodless and can be done bluntly to some extent. The pancreatic mass can be palpated between the surgeon's thumb and index/middle fingers. This allows the surgeon to confirm the absence of vascular involvement and resectability of the mass.
2. The gallbladder is dissected in a dome down fashion and the junction of the cystic duct with the common bile duct is exposed.
3. The bile duct is divided with an electrocautery device proximal to its junction with the cystic duct. The gall bladder can be removed en bloc with the main specimen or can be removed separately.
4. The lesser sac is opened by dividing the gastrocolic ligament. The inferior border of the pancreas is dissected until the inferior mesenteric vein is identified. A tunnel is created behind the neck of the pancreas over the inferior mesenteric vein.
5. A portal dissection is performed, removing all nodal tissue from the portal triad. The gastroduodenal artery is exposed and ligated close to its take-off. Prior to ligating the gastroduodenal artery, it is important to test clamp and confirm the flow to the proper hepatic artery is preserved.
6. A tunnel is then created at the level of the pancreas neck, between the posterior surface of the pancreas and

the anterior surface of the portal vein. Typically this segment of the portal vein has no tributaries and can be completed with minimal blood loss. However, this dissection can be challenging in those patients with prior episodes of pancreatitis or a large tumor invading the portal vein.

7. Once the tunnel is created, a penrose or a vessel loop is passed around the level of the neck of the pancreas.

8. In a standard Whipple, the antrum is transected proximal to the pylorus whereas in a pylorus-preserving Whipple, the duodenum is divided just beyond the pylorus.

9. The proximal jejunum is then divided about 10 cm distal to the ligament of Treitz.

10. The mesentery is divided with the help of an advanced energy device and the jejunal limb is passed behind the ligament of Treitz.

11. The pancreatic parenchyma is then divided with an electrocautery device while some tension is held on the penrose. Any bleeding from the pancreatic parenchyma can be controlled with stay sutures.

12. The uncinate process and the head of the pancreas are dissected off the superior mesenteric artery and the portal vein using an energy device.

13. The specimen is delivered off the field and hemostasis is achieved.

Reconstruction

1. There are several ways to perform the pancreatico-jejunostomy reconstruction.

2. The cut end of the jejunum is passed in a retrocolic fashion right of the middle colic vessels.

3. The jejunum loop is placed in an end-to-side configuration in order to start the pancreaticojejunostomy.

Pancreaticojejunostomy:

Duct-to-mucosa Technique

1. A posterior row of interrupted non-absorbable sutures is placed taking seromuscular bites on the jejunum and the posterior capsule of the pancreas.
2. An enterotomy is made on the jejunum. Using a fine absorbable suture, the duct to mucosa anastomosis is performed, completing the posterior row first and moving to the anterior row. It is important to note that depending on the size of the duct, between 4 and 10 interrupted sutures are placed. An 8 Fr pediatric feeding tube is sometimes left in place to keep the anastomosis patent.
3. The anterior row of non-absorbable sutures are placed taking seromuscular bites on the jejunum side and including the anterior capsule of the pancreas.

Invagination Technique

In cases where the pancreatic duct is really small (<2–3 mm), this technique is chosen. The pancreas is anchored to the jejunal limb taking two full thickness bites through the jejunal wall at the superior and inferior border. The open jejunal end is then sutured to the pancreas capsule with interrupted non absorbable sutures.

Hepaticojejunostomy:

1. An enterotomy is made a few cm distal to the pancreaticojejunostomy.
2. A series of absorbable interrupted sutures are placed making sure that full thickness bites are taken on the jejunal side.
3. The sutures are all placed without being tied in order to facilitate visualization and the posterior row is completed and tied first, followed by the anterior row.

Gastrojejunostomy/duodenojejunostomy

1. Jejunal limb is brought in an antecolic fashion distal to the hepaticojejunostomy.

2. A side-to-side gastrojejunostomy is fashioned in case of a standard Whipple and end-to-side duodenojejunostomy is fashioned in case of a pylorus-preserving Whipple. This can be performed handsewn or by using a surgical stapling device.

3. Careful hemostasis is achieved and the abdomen is irrigated.

4. Two drains are placed spanning the hepaticojejunostomy and pancreaticojejunostomy.

5. The abdomen is closed in the standard fashion (Fig. 28.1).

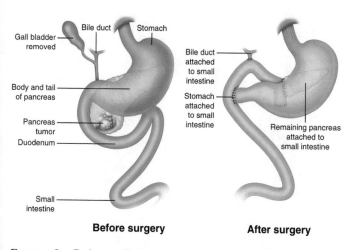

Gall bladder removed

Bile duct   Stomach

Body and tail of pancreas

Pancreas tumor

Duodenum

Small intestine

Bile duct attached to small intestine

Stomach attached to small intestine

Remaining pancreas attached to small intestine

Before surgery

After surgery

Figure 28.1 Before and after pancreadicoduodenectomy

Part VII
Biliary System

Chapter 29
Laparoscopic Cholecystectomy

Efstathios Karamanos

Overview

- Hasson or veress needle entry
- Identify gallbladder, and retract cranially and laterally
- Take down peritoneal attachments
- Identify and isolate cystic duct
- Identify and isolate cystic artery
- Confirm critical view prior to ligating and dividing duct and artery
- Dissect gallbladder off liver
- Intraop cholangiogram if indicated

Clinical Pearls

- Start dissection laterally as there are no critical structures there
- Critical view consists of:

  - Two and only two structures going into gallbladder
  - Cystic plate visualized posterior to gallbladder
  - Hepatocystic triangle cleared off

E. Karamanos (✉)
Plastic and Reconstructive Surgery, UT Health San Antonio, San Antonio, TX, USA

© Springer Nature Switzerland AG 2020   179
E. Karamanos (ed.), *Common Surgeries Made Easy*,
https://doi.org/10.1007/978-3-030-41350-7_29

- Callot's Triangle

  - Cystic duct
  - Common hepatic duct
  - Inferior edge of liver
  - Contains the cystic artery

- CBD stone on cholangiogram

  - Give glucagon and flush biliary system to attempt to dislodge
  - Laparoscopic basket retrieval
  - Laparoscopic CBD exploration
  - Open CBD exploration
  - Transduodenal ductotomy if impacted distal CBD stone

- Postop hyperbilirubinemia and leukocytosis

  - Ultrasound to assess for biloma
  - HIDA scan to assess for bile leak

- Bile Leak Treatment

  - ERCP and stent placement if cystic duct stump leak +/− IR drain
  - Common bile duct exploration if CBD injury with closure over T-tube

Patient Placement

Supine with arms out. Place foot board because patient will be in reverse Trendelenburg position for most of the operation. The foot pedal for the electrocautery device goes to the left of the patient. The patient does not need a nasogastric tube. If you expect a long operative time then a Foley might be indicated, but generally, there is no need for a Foley catheter. Prep the patient with chlorhexidine prep from the nipples to the pubic symphysis.

Anesthesia

General anesthesia.

Operative Steps

1. Incise the skin using a transverse infraumbilical or supra-umbilical incision. On the techniques of how to enter the abdomen refer to the chapter: entering the abdomen.
2. Once you have gained access to the peritoneal cavity, insufflate and inspect with a 5 mm, 30° scope.
3. Proceed with placing the rest of the ports: 10 mm port subxiphoid, and two 5 mm ports at the right lateral abdominal wall along the costal margin. When placing the 10 mm port, take care to enter right to the falciform ligament as this will make dissection easier.
4. Insert two non – traumatic graspers at the lateral 5 mm ports and a Maryland dissector at the 10 mm port at the xiphoid process.
5. With one of the non – traumatic graspers, grab the fundus of the gallbladder and push cephalad and towards the right shoulder above the liver.
6. With the other non – traumatic grasper grab the infundibulum and retract lateral towards the abdominal wall. This exposes the hepatocystic triangle.
7. With the hook cautery, incise the peritoneum that is encasing the gallbladder. Flip the infundibulum medially so that the lateral peritoneal dissection happens first. Continue incising the peritoneum cephalad for at least 2/3 of the gallbladder wall if possible.
8. Retract the gallbladder infundibulum lateral and continue incising the peritoneum medially in the same fashion. Be cognizant of the cystic artery or any replaced anatomy.

9. Using your Maryland dissector, dissect the cystic duct first by identifying where the infundibulum becomes the cystic duct. The safest and easiest way to identify it is by dissecting into the triangle, first lateral and then proceed with the medial dissection.

10. Once the cystic duct has been identified, look for the cystic artery posteromedial to the duct and isolate it. A laparoscopic right angle is often helpful.

11. Obtain the critical view of safety: hepatocystic triangle cleared of any fibrous of fatty tissue, the lower one third of the gallbladder is separated from the liver to expose the lower part of the cystic plate and two and only two structures are seen entering the gallbladder (Fig. 29.1).

12. Clip the duct first: using a laparoscopic clip applier, place two clip proximally and one distally and transect the duct between.

13. Repeat the same process for the cystic artery.

14. Once you have verified that there is not a replaced left hepatic artery then proceed with the dissection of the gallbladder from the cystic plate. You may use a spatula or a hook for that part.

15. Insert the laparoscopic specimen retrieval bag through the 10 mm port and place the gallbladder in the bag. Remove the bag through the incision by first removing the port. If you need to stretch the fascia of the incision, you may do so by using a Kelly clamp.

16. Once the specimen is out, ensure you have good hemostasis and there is no bile spillage. If you have stones or bile spillage use a laparoscopic suction.

17. Close the fascia of the 10 mm port using a 0 Vicryl suture on a UR needle. In a figure of eight fashion.

18. Close the skin on all the ports with 4-0 monocryl suture in a subcuticular fashion.

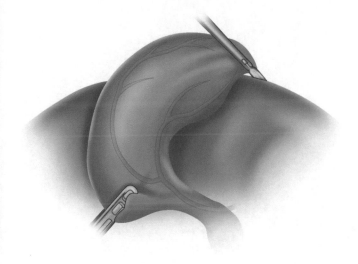

Figure 29.1 The critical view of safety

Chapter 30
Open Cholecystectomy

Hassan Nasser and Efstathios Karamanos

Overview

- Falciform ligament taken down
- Gallbladder grasped and dissection started dome down towards infundibulum/cystic duct junction
- Cystic duct and artery identified, isolated, and ligated
- Cholangiogram if indicated

Clinical Pearls

- Callot's Triangle

    - Cystic duct
    - Common hepatic duct
    - Inferior edge of liver
    - Contains the cystic artery

- Cystic artery branches off right hepatic artery

H. Nasser
Department of General Surgery, Henry Ford Hospital/Wayne State University, Detroit, MI, USA

E. Karamanos (✉)
Plastic and Reconstructive Surgery, UT Health San Antonio, San Antonio, TX, USA

© Springer Nature Switzerland AG 2020
E. Karamanos (ed.), *Common Surgeries Made Easy*,
https://doi.org/10.1007/978-3-030-41350-7_30

- Blood supply to CBD runs at 3 o'clock and 9 o'clock position
- CBD stone on cholangiogram

  - Give glucagon and flush biliary system to attempt to dislodge
  - Open CBD exploration
  - Transduodenal ductotomy if impacted distal CBD stone

- Postop hyperbilirubinemia and leukocytosis

  - Ultrasound to assess for biloma
  - HIDA scan to assess for bile leak

- Bile Leak Treatment

  - ERCP and stent placement if cystic duct stump leak +/− IR drain
  - Common bile duct exploration if CBD injury with closure over T-tube

Patient Placement

Place the patient supine.
  Arms out.
  No Foley is required.
  Prep the abdomen with chlorhexidine.
  A nasogastric tube is placed to decompress the stomach.

Anesthesia

General anesthesia is required.

Operative Steps

1. A right subcostal incision is made two finger breadths below the costal margin from the midline to the anterior axillary line. An upper midline laparotomy can be used in some cases.

2. The incision is carried down through the subcutaneous tissue, Scarpa's fascia, external oblique, internal oblique, and transversus abdominis.

3. The peritoneum is identified and grasped between two forceps and then incised sharply using Metzenbaum scissors.

4. The falciform ligament is identified and divided between silk ties.

5. The abdomen is explored.

6. Any adhesions to the gallbladder are taken down sharply or using an electrocautery device.

7. A Bookwalter retractor is placed to assist with retraction (Fig. 30.1).

8. If the gallbladder is acutely inflamed and distended, aspiration of gallbladder contents may be necessary to facilitate its manipulation.

9. The fundus of the gallbladder is grasped with a Kelly clamp and dissected of the liver using electrocautery.

10. At the neck of the gallbladder, the cystic duct and artery are carefully identified. These two structures are divided between two clips or silk ties. The common bile duct is palpated to ensure that there are no retained stones in the duct.

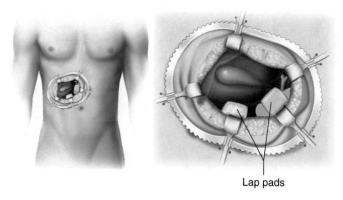

Lap pads

Figure 30.1 Subcostal incision for open cholecystectomy

11. If there is any difficulty identifying the cystic structures or there is a concern for a retained stone, a cholangiogram can be performed.

12. The surgical bed is irrigated and suctioned. Hemostasis is ensured.

13. *A drain is placed in the gallbladder fossa if there is concern of a biliary leak.*

14. The wound is closed in two running layers using a #1 PDS suture. The first layer includes the peritoneum, transversus abdominis, and internal oblique laterally, and posterior rectus sheath medially. The second layer includes the external oblique laterally and anterior rectus sheath medially.

15. The Scarpa's fascia is then closed with an interrupted 3–0 Vicryl suture.

16. The skin is closed with staples. *Leave the skin open if there is significant contamination or an abscess is present.*

Part VIII
Hernia

Chapter 31
Inguinal Hernia Repair – Open Tissue Repair (Bassini)

Efstathios Karamanos

Overview

- Skin incision made 2 cm superior and lateral to pubic symphysis extending towards ASIS
- Dissect to external oblique fascia, and incise
- Protect ilioinguinal nerve, and retract external oblique fascia to expose spermatic cord/round ligament
- Encircle spermatic cord
- Dissect cremasteric muscle fibers off spermatic cord and assess for indirect and direct hernias
- Reduce indirect hernia if present
- Primary repair of direct hernia

Clinical Pearls

- Indirect hernia is anteromedial to spermatic cord, as result of patent processus vaginalis
    - Lateral to Hasselbach's triangle

E. Karamanos (✉)
Plastic and Reconstructive Surgery, UT Health San Antonio,
San Antonio, TX, USA

© Springer Nature Switzerland AG 2020
E. Karamanos (ed.), *Common Surgeries Made Easy*,
https://doi.org/10.1007/978-3-030-41350-7_31

- Direct hernias are due to weakness of inguinal floor, made up of transversalis fascia

  - Within Hasslebach's triangle

- Hasselbach's triangle made up of

  - Linea semilunaris
  - Inguinal ligament
  - Inferior Epigastric Vessels

- Ilioinguinal nerve innervates upper scrotum, root of penis or labia majora

  - Most commonly injured nerve in open repair

- Contents of spermatic cord

  - Testicular artery
  - Pampiniform plexus
  - Genital branch of genitofemoral nerve
  - Vas deferens

Patient Placement

Supine, arms out, no need for a Foley catheter, chlorhexidine prep. The genitalia can be prepped into the field but they usually are not.

Anesthesia

Sedation with local anesthesia or general are acceptable based on patient's preference and peri-operative risk factors.

Local Anesthesia

1. Identify the Anterior Superior Iliac Spine (ASIS). Create a wheel with local anesthetic about 2 cm superior and anterior to the ASIS.

2. With the needle in 90° from the skin insert the abdominal wall until the needle is between the external oblique aponeurosis and the internal oblique aponeurosis. Inject some cc of a local anesthetic.

3. Identify the pubic symphysis. Insert the needle in 45° until the needle touches the bone. Insert some cc of a local anesthetic.

4. With the needle in about 10° from the skin insert at where the skin incision will be and anesthetize the skin with several cc of a local anesthetic.

5. Replicate the same process to anesthetize the same area but deeper including the subcutaneous tissue.

6. Identify the midline and move lateral about 1 cm. Inject the subcutaneous tissue several times starting from the pubic symphysis and moving cephalad until you have reached the umbilicus.

7. (Later) When you have dissected the spermatic cord, inject a small amount of local anesthesia to the cremasteric muscles.

Landmarks for the Skin Incision

Identify the pubic symphysis. Move laterally and anterior about 2 cm. This is where the external ring approximately is.

Feel for the femoral artery pulse. The internal ring is at the same cephalad-caudad line.

The iliopubic tract (Poupart's ligament or inguinal ligament) connects the ASIS to the pubic symphysis.

The skin incision should adequately expose the internal and external rings.

Operative Steps

1. Incise the skin.

2. Dissect down to the Camper's fascia. Some crossing veins can be either cauterized or free tied depending on the size.

3. Dissect through the Scarpa's fascia.
4. Continue dissecting deep until the external oblique aponeurosis is identified.
5. Identify the external ring close to the pubic symphysis. Notice a change in the quality of the external oblique aponeurosis medially. Notice the Y shaped area. This is where the incision will be.
6. With the 15 blade, make a 0.5 cm incision on the fascia following the direction of the fibers (from the ASIS to the pubic symphysis).
7. Using Metzenbaum scissors slide underneath the incised fascia and extend the incision towards the external ring. Open the external ring. Extend your incision towards the ASIS using the same technique. THE ILIOINGUINAL NERVE LIES UNDERNEATH; AVOID INJURING IT!!!!
8. Use two Kelly clamps to grasp the incised ends of the external oblique aponeurosis.
9. Using fingers, create a space between the external oblique and the conjoined tendon.
10. Identify the spermatic cord in males and the round ligament in females. Encircle the spermatic cord with a penrose drain.
11. Assess for the presence of an indirect hernia. This will be anterior and medial to the spermatic cord.
12. Using two Debakey pick –ups, dissect the hernia sac free from the spermatic cord down to the level of the internal ring.
13. Allow the hernia sac to reduce and return to the peritoneum. If the internal ring is too lax, it can be reapproximated with a permanent suture in a figure of eight fashion.
14. Assess for the presence of a direct hernia.
15. Grab the conjoined tendon using one Allis clamp.
16. Approximate the conjoined tendon to the inguinal ligament using a 0 Ethibond suture. Avoid injury to the vein by taking superficial bites to the inguinal ligament. Every bite should be on a different level on the inguinal ligament to avoid recurrence.

17. Assess for a tension free repair. If tension is a concern, perform a relaxing incision.
18. Close the external oblique aponeurosis with a 2–0 Vicryl suture in a continuous fashion.
19. Close the Scarpa's fascia with a 3–0 Vicryl suture in a continuous fashion.
20. Close the skin with a 4–0 Vicryl suture in a subcuticular fashion (Fig. 31.1).

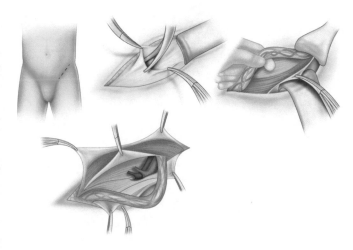

FIGURE 31.1 Inguinal anatomy

Chapter 32
Open Inginual Hernia Repair – Lichtenstein Repair

Jaclyn Yracheta, Claire Gerall, Mallory Wampler, Michael Sippel, and Efstathios Karamanos

Overview

- Skin incision made 2 cm superior and lateral to pubic symphysis extending towards ASIS
- Dissect to external oblique fascia, and incise
- Protect ilioinguinal nerve, and retract external oblique fascia to expose spermatic cord/round ligament
- Encircle spermatic cord
- Dissect cremasteric muscle fibers off spermatic cord and assess for indirect and direct hernias
- Reduce indirect hernia if present
- Mesh repair of direct and indirect hernia

J. Yracheta · C. Gerall · M. Wampler · M. Sippel
Department of Surgery, UT Health San Antonio, San Antonio, TX, USA

E. Karamanos (✉)
Plastic and Reconstructive Surgery, UT Health San Antonio, San Antonio, TX, USA

© Springer Nature Switzerland AG 2020
E. Karamanos (ed.), *Common Surgeries Made Easy*,
https://doi.org/10.1007/978-3-030-41350-7_32

Clinical Pearls

- Indirect hernia is anteromedial to spermatic cord, as result of patent processus vaginalis

  - Lateral to Hasselbach's triangle

- Direct hernias are due to weakness of inguinal floor, made up of transversalis fascia

  - Within Hasslebach's triangle

- Hasselbach's triangle made up of

  - Linea semilunaris
  - Inguinal ligament
  - Inferior Epigastric Vessels

- Ilioinguinal nerve innervates upper scrotum, root of penis or labia majora

  - Most commonly injured nerve in open repair

- Contents of spermatic cord

  - Testicular artery
  - Pampiniform plexus
  - Genital branch of genitofemoral nerve
  - Vas deferens

Patient Placement

The patient should be placed in supine position. Verify the location of the pathology and the appropriate groin should be prepped and draped in the usual sterile fashion.

Anesthesia

Although general anesthesia is most commonly used, spinal or local anesthesia with sedation can be used as well. See previous chapter for the steps for local anesthetic administration.

Operative Steps

Follow steps from 1 to 14 from the Bassini repair. Once all those steps have been completed, perform the following steps:

1. An appropriately sized, flat, polypropylene mesh with a lateral keyhole should be used.
2. Using a 2–0 or 3–0 nonabsorbable suture, fix the mesh to the pubic tubercle in an interrupted fashion. Be sure to place the suture into the periosteum and back through the mesh. The mesh should extend 2 cm medially past the pubic tubercle to avoid medial recurrence.
3. Using a 2–0 or 3–0 nonabsorbable suture in an interrupted fashion, fix the mesh inferiorly to the shelving edge of the inguinal ligament. For the first 3–4 sutures, do not tie initially, instead secure with a hemostat to assess mesh alignment before securing the mesh in place. The sutures should be placed about 7–10 mm apart. Carry the inferior suture line 2 cm lateral to the internal ring. Care should be taken to avoid underlying structures (Fig. 32.1).
4. Once the inferior suture line joining the mesh and the inguinal ligament is mostly complete, the two mesh tails of the keyhole can be joined and secured using the same suture.
5. Next, the superior suture line is made by joining the mesh to the conjoint tendon using 2–0 or 3–0 nonabsorbable suture in an interrupted fashion. Carry the suture line 2 cm lateral to the internal ring.
6. Assess the internal ring, it should accommodate the tip of a Kelly hemostat. A single suture can be placed lateral to the cord to tighten the ring as needed.

    (a) In females: Completely close the internal ring.

7. Ensure hemostasis using an electrocautery device and remove the penrose drain.
8. Close the aponeurosis of the external oblique in a running fashion with a 2–0 Vicryl suture. Take care to avoid catching the ilioinguinal nerve in the suture line.

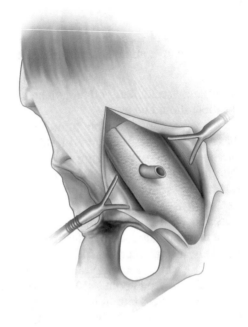

FIGURE 32.1 Placement of mesh

9. Close the Scarpa's fascia and the subcutaneous tissue with interrupted 3–0 Vicryl sutures.

10. Administer a field block for local anesthesia: Inject a local anesthetic along the skin incision. Additionally, a fascial injection should be given 2 cm medial and cephalad from the anterior superior iliac spine (ASIS) to block the ilio-inguinal nerve.

11. Close the skin in a subcuticular manner with a 4–0 Monocryl suture. Apply a sterile dressing.

12. Following the skin closure and dressing application, gently pull the testis to its anatomic position.

Disclaimer
The views expressed are those of the [author(s)] [presenter(s)] and do not reflect the official views or policy of the Department of Defense or its Component.

Chapter 33
Open Femoral Hernia Repair – McVay

Jaclyn Yracheta, Claire Gerall, Mallory Wampler, Michael Sippel, and Efstathios Karamanos

Overview

- Skin incision made 2 cm superior and lateral to pubic symphysis extending towards ASIS
- Dissect to external oblique fascia, and incise
- Protect ilioinguinal nerve, and retract external oblique fascia to expose spermatic cord/round ligament
- Encircle spermatic cord
- Dissect cremasteric muscle fibers off spermatic cord and assess for indirect and direct hernias
- Expose Cooper's ligament, and assess mobility
- Make relaxing incision in anterior rectus sheath
- Primarily close Cooper's ligament to Conjoint Tendon to level of femoral vessels
- Transition Stitch at femoral vessels to primarily close Conjoint Tendon to Inguinal Ligament
- Tighten internal ring if indicated (obliterate in females)

J. Yracheta · C. Gerall · M. Wampler · M. Sippel
Department of Surgery, UT Health San Antonio, San Antonio, TX, USA

E. Karamanos (✉)
Plastic and Reconstructive Surgery, UT Health San Antonio, San Antonio, TX, USA

© Springer Nature Switzerland AG 2020
E. Karamanos (ed.), *Common Surgeries Made Easy*,
https://doi.org/10.1007/978-3-030-41350-7_33

Clinical Pearls

- Femoral hernias are more common in females
- Need relaxing incision to obtain tension-free repair

Patient Placement

The patient should be placed in supine position. Verify the location of the pathology and the appropriate groin should be prepped and draped in the usual sterile fashion.

Anesthesia

Although general anesthesia is most commonly used, spinal or local anesthesia with sedation can be used as well.

Operative Steps

Follow steps from 1 to 14 from the Bassini repair. Once all those steps have been completed, perform the following steps:

1. Expose the Cooper's ligament by sharp and blunt dissection.
2. Identify the conjoint tendon and grasp it with an Allis clamp to assess the quality and mobility to the Cooper's ligament.
3. Using an electrocautery device, make a relaxing incision in the anterior rectus sheath, medial and superior to the conjoint tendon. Again, assess the mobility of the conjoint tendon to the Cooper's ligament, which should reach easily without tension.

4. Use a 2–0 or 3–0 nonabsorbable suture in an interrupted fashion to suture the conjoint tend to the Cooper's ligament, beginning at the pubic tubercle and progressing laterally until you reach the femoral vessels.

5. At the medial aspect of the femoral vein, place a transition stitch to incorporate the conjoint tendon, Cooper's ligament and the anterior femoral sheath. The remaining sutures should be placed between the conjoint tendon and the inguinal ligament laterally to the level of the internal ring. Care should be taken when suturing to avoid the femoral vessels.

6. Assess the internal ring, it should accommodate the tip of a Kelly hemostat. A single suture can be placed lateral to the cord to tighten the ring as needed.

   (a) In females: Completely close the internal ring.

7. Ensure for hemostasis using electrocautery and remove the penrose drain.

8. Close the aponeurosis of the external oblique in a running fashion with a 2–0 Vicryl suture. Take care to avoid catching the ilioinguinal nerve in the suture line.

9. Close Scarpa's fascia and subcutaneous tissue with interrupted 3–0 Vicryl sutures.

10. Administer a field block for local anesthesia: Inject a local anesthetic along the skin incision. Additionally, a fascial injection should be given 2 cm medial and cephalad from the anterior superior iliac spine (ASIS) to block the ilioinguinal nerve.

11. Close the skin in a subcuticular manner with a 4–0 Monocryl suture. Apply a sterile dressing.

12. Following the skin closure and dressing application, gently pull the testis to its anatomic position (Fig. 33.1).

Disclaimer
The views expressed are those of the [author(s)] [presenter(s)] and do not reflect the official views or policy of the Department of Defense or its Component.

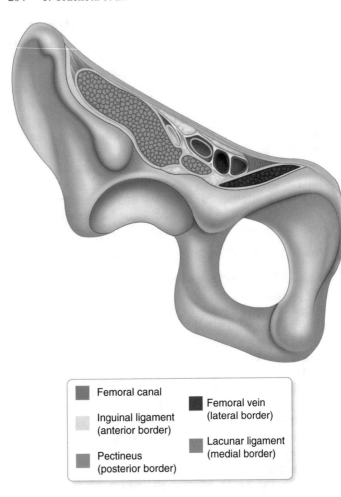

Femoral canal

Inguinal ligament
(anterior border)

Pectineus
(posterior border)

Femoral vein
(lateral border)

Lacunar ligament
(medial border)

FIGURE 33.1 Anatomy of the femoral canal

Chapter 34
Laparoscopic Totally Extraperitoneal (TEP) Inguinal Hernia Repair

Marianne Franco

Overview

- An infraumbilical incision is made and the rectus sheath is incised, allowing access to the preperitoneal space. A balloon is used to separate the peritoneum from the rectus muscle, creating the working space. Anatomical landmarks are used to identify the indirect, direct and femoral spaces. Herniating tissue is reduced as well as the indirect sac. Mesh is tacked into place to cover the direct, indirect and femoral spaces.

Clinical Pearls

- Femoral Canal Borders
    - Anterosuperiorly by the inguinal ligament
    - Posteriorly by the pectineal ligament
    - Medially by the lacunar ligament
    - Laterally by the femoral vein

M. Franco (✉)

Henry Ford West Bloomfield Hospital, West Bloomfield, MI, USA

e-mail: mfranco1@hfhs.org

© Springer Nature Switzerland AG 2020

E. Karamanos (ed.), *Common Surgeries Made Easy*,

https://doi.org/10.1007/978-3-030-41350-7_34

- Corona Mortis

  - "Crown of Death"
  - Vascular anastomosis between the external iliac or inferior epigastric vessels and the obturator vessels

- Triangle of Doom

  - Borders are Vas deferens, testicular artery, and peritoneal fold
  - External Iliac Artery and Vein course through here

- Triangle of Pain

  - V-shaped area bounded by iliopubic tract and spermatic vessels
  - Contains lateral femoral cutaneous, femoral, and genitofemoral nerves

- Lateral Femoral Cutaneous Nerve - innervates skin of lateral thigh

  - Most commonly injured nerve in lap hernia repair

- Hesselbach's triangle made up of

  - Lateral border of the rectus abdominus muscle
  - Inguinal ligament
  - Inferior Epigastric Vessels

- Contents of spermatic cord

  - Testicular artery
  - Pampiniform plexus
  - Genital branch of genitofemoral nerve
  - Vas deferens
  - Parasympathetic and sympathetics nerves
  - Lymphatic vessels
  - Cremasteric artery
  - Artery of the ductus deferens

Patient Placement

Supine with both arms tucked if performing bilateral repair, opposite arm if unilateral. A Foley catheter placement is surgeon dependent. Prep the skin with chloraprep. The surgeon and the assistant stand on the side opposite of the hernia being addressed.

Anesthesia

General endotracheal anesthesia.

Operative Steps

1. Make an infraumbilical incision biased toward the side of the hernia being repaired. If performing bilateral hernia repair, bias the incision toward the side of the larger hernia.
2. Bluntly dissect down to the anterior rectus sheath, NOT the midline.
3. Incise the anterior rectus sheath horizontally, exposing the rectus muscle. The fascial incision should be approximately 12 mm.
4. Find the medial edge of the rectus muscle and place an S or Army-Navy retractor under the belly of the rectus muscle, exposing the posterior rectus sheath.
5. While lifting the belly of the rectus muscle with the retractor, insert the balloon dissector into the preperitoneal space which is below the rectus muscle and above the posterior rectus sheath. Keep the balloon dissector parallel to the abdominal wall as you advance the balloon to the pubic tubercle. There should be little to no resistance while advancing.

6. Insert the 0° camera and inflate the balloon dissector. Keep the balloon inflated for 30-60 seconds to achieve hemostasis of small vessels.
7. Deflate the balloon dissector and remove.
8. Inflate the port balloon and insufflate the preperitoneal space to 12–15 mm Hg CO_2.
9. Switch to the 30° camera.
10. Place a 5 mm port in the midline, two fingerbreadths above the pubic tubercle.
11. Place a second 5 mm port in the midline, halfway between the 12 mm infraumbilical port and the 5 mm suprapubic port.
12. Identify any readily visible anatomical landmarks for orientation, most often the epigastric vessels.
13. Start the dissection with blunt instruments (Kitners or atraumatic graspers) lateral to the epigastrics, pushing the avelolar tissue down as you slowly approach the lateral pelvic wall.
14. As the alvelolar tissue is dissected away, the peritoneal edge should become visible. Follow the peritoneal edge toward the pelvis and and this will help you identify the location of the spermatic cord. The spermatic cord will enter the internal ring, lateral to the epigastric vessels (Fig. 34.1).
15. Once the spermatic cord is identified, continue the blunt dissection of the alvelolar tissue more inferiorly and medially, exposing the femoral vein, Cooper's ligament and pubic tubercle.
16. Now that the anatomic landmarks are exposed, orient yourself and identify the femoral, direct and indirect spaces and address each area.
17. If the inferior edge of the peritoneum is readily visible on the spermatic cord, an indirect hernia is not present. The peritoneum, however, should still be gently dissected away from the cord and pushed back to the level of the umbilicus.

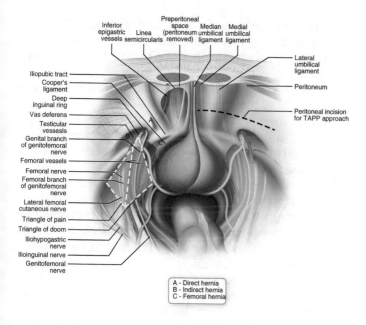

FIGURE 34.1 Anatomy of the inguinal region

18. If the peritoneal edge enters the internal ring (lateral to the epigastric vessels) alongside the spermatic cord, an indirect hernia is present. Gently grab the peritoneum with an atraumatic grasper and place cephalad traction with one hand. With the other hand, dissect away the spermatic cord structures. Use scissors to cut any adhesions only after definitively identifying the vas deferens and spermatic vessels. Dissection must continue until the inferior edge of the peritoneum is identified and pushed back to the level of the umbilicus.

19. If a hole is made in the peritoneum during dissection, it can be closed with 5 mm clip applier. If visualization is impaired from "competing pneumo's" insert a Veress needle in the peritoneal cavity to evacuate the air.

20. Examine the lateral edge of the spermatic cord for an avascular cord lipoma and reduce.

21. Identify if direct and femoral hernias are present. Reduce any herniating tissue with gentle traction. The hernias are fully reduced when all the tissue has fallen below Cooper's ligament.
22. Roll the mesh and insert it into the preperitoneal space through the camera port.
23. Orient the mesh correctly. The medial edge should be just lateral to the pubic tubercle and should cover the direct, femoral and indirect spaces. The inferior edge should fall just below Cooper's.
24. Fixate the mesh with an absorbable spiral tacker medially on Cooper's ligament (beware of corona mortis and femoral vein), superiorly on the rectus muscle (beware of epigastric vessels) and laterally on the pelvic sidewall (avoid Triangle of Pain). Other options of fixation include fibrin glue or no fixation at all.
25. Examine cavity for hemostasis.
26. Under direct visualization, withdraw the 5 mm ports. Deflate the pneumoperitoneum, making sure the mesh does not fold and "clam-shell" upon collapse of the preperitoneal space.
27. Close the fascial incision and skin incisions with absorbable sutures.

Chapter 35
Laparoscopic Inguinal Hernia Repair – TAPP

Puraj Patel

Overview

- Hasson or Veress needle into abdomen periumbilically
- Place 2 more 5 mm ports one to right, and one to left of periumbilical port, and upsize periumbilical port to 12 mm port
- Using lap scissors and Maryland dissector, create horizontal window in peritoneal 2 cm inferior to umbilicus
- Dissect peritoneum off abdominal wall to expose pubic tubercle and Cooper's ligament
- Start dissection lateral to epigastric vessels, pushing down alveolar tissue exposing peritoneal edge
- Expose spermatic cord, Cooper's ligament, and pubic tubercle
- Identify femoral, direct, and indirect hernia spaces
- Dissect indirect hernia sac off spermatic cord if present
- Reduce any herniating tissue from direct or femoral hernia if present
- Tac mesh in place
- Close peritoneal window with sutures or tacs

P. Patel (✉)
Henry Ford West Bloomfield Hospital, West Bloomfield, MI, USA
e-mail: ppatel13@hfhs.org

© Springer Nature Switzerland AG 2020
E. Karamanos (ed.), *Common Surgeries Made Easy*,
https://doi.org/10.1007/978-3-030-41350-7_35

Clinical Pearls

- Triangle of Doom

  - Borders are Vas deferens, testicular artery, and peritoneal fold
  - External Iliac Artery and Vein course through here

- Triangle of Pain

  - V-shaped area bounded by iliopubic tract and spermatic vessels
  - Contains lateral femoral cutaneous, femoral, and genitofemoral nerves

- Lateral Femoral Cutaneous Nerve - innervates skin of lateral thigh

  - Most commonly injured nerve in lap hernia repair

- Hasselbach's triangle made up of

  - Linea semilunaris
  - Inguinal ligament
  - Inferior Epigastric Vessels

- Contents of spermatic cord

  - Testicular artery
  - Pampiniform plexus
  - Genital branch of genitofemoral nerve
  - Vas deferens

Patient Placement

Supine with both arms tucked. A Foley catheter placement is surgeon dependent. Prep the skin with chloroprep and include the genitalia if there is a large scrotal component to the hernia sac. When repairing a right inguinal hernia, the surgeon stands to the left of the patient facing the feet and the assistant is on the right of the patient, also facing the feet. When repairing a left inguinal hernia, the surgeon stands to the right of the patient facing the feet and the assistant is on the left of the patient, also facing the feet. The monopolar foot pedal is placed on the surgeon's side. If bilateral inguinal hernias are present, the surgeon and assistant first approach one side in this manner and then switch sides to repair the contralateral hernia.

Anesthesia

General endotracheal anesthesia is required. Using local anesthesia is also preferred for the laparoscopic port sites prior to skin incision.

Landmarks and Skin Incisions

Identifying the ASIS and pubic tubercle prior to incision is prudent. Typically three port sites are used for a TAPP inguinal hernia repair. An infraumbilical 12 mm circumlinear incision is used. Two additional 5 mm port sites are located laterally left and right to the initial incision approximately 8–10 cm away, at the mid clavicular line.

Once pneumoperitoneum is established and a diagnostic laparoscopy is performed, the following key structures should be identified:

- Median and medial umbilical folds
- Epigastric vessels
- Vas deferens and spermatic vessels (male)
- Iliac vessels
- Hernia defect

Operative Steps (Example of Right Inguinal Hernia Repair)

1. Create a 12 mm circumlinear infraumbilical incision. Dissect down to the anterior fascia and the umbilical stalk.
2. Use a Kocher clamp to secure the base of the umbilical stalk. Use a second Kocher clamp to secure slightly caudal to the first clamp.
3. Using a 15-blade scalpel, incise the anterior fascia.
4. Use a Kelly clamp to bluntly enter the abdominal cavity through the peritoneum.
5. Insert a 5 mm trocar (without the obturator) into the peritoneal cavity.
6. Insufflate the abdomen to 15 mmHg of CO_2.
7. Perform a diagnostic laparoscopy with a 30° angled 5 mm laparoscope, examining each of the 4 abdominal quadrants.
8. Place a 5 mm laparoscopic port approximately 8–10 cm right lateral to the umbilical incision.
9. Move the camera to the right lateral 5 mm trocar.
10. Switch out the initial access 5 mm trocar to a 12 mm trocar.
11. Place the final 5 mm laparoscopic port approximately 8–10 cm left lateral to the umbilical incision.
12. Begin with laparoscopic scissors in the umbilical (12 mm) trocar with the monopolar cord attached and a Maryland grasper/dissector in the left lateral (5 mm) trocar.
13. Create a horizontal incision in the peritoneum 2 cm below the level of the umbilicus beginning at the medial umbilical ligament towards the ASIS.
14. Using a combination of the laparoscopic scissors and blunt graspers, carefully dissect the peritoneum away from the abdominal wall. This is usually accomplished by grasping the cut edge of the peritoneum and retracting it cephalad and posterior.

15. Beginning at the medial aspect of the peritoneal flap allows identification of the pubic tubercle and Cooper's ligament. For large direct hernias dissection across midline is prudent for mesh overlap.

16. Remove any fat in Hasselbach triangle to identify direct hernia defects.

17. Dissection between the Cooper's ligament and the bladder is performed, allowing the medial and inferior edges of the mesh to lay flat towards the space of Retzius.

18. Dissection between Cooper's ligament and the iliac vein is performed to identify a femoral hernia defect.

19. Parietalize the cord structures to clearly identify and reduce an indirect hernia sac. The cord structures should lay flat against the pelvic wall. The psoas muscle and iliac vessels should be identifiable.

20. At times, long indirect sacs in scrotal hernias can be transected. The peritoneal defect should be closed.

21. Identify and reduce cord lipomas. These are usually lateral to the cord structures.

22. Dissection lateral to the hernia is performed beyond the ASIS, sweeping posterior and cephalad, for lateral mesh placement.

23. Minimum mesh size should be 15×10 cm, although typically larger piece may be necessary to cover the entire myopectineal orifice. May also use a pre-formed right- or left-sided mesh.

24. Grasp the medial edge of the chosen mesh and insert through the 12 mm trocar and place the grasper on the pubic bone.

25. Use the left lateral 5 mm trocar and another blunt grasper to grasp the lateral edge of the mesh and place it laterally in the pocket.

26. Once the mesh position is confirmed, the mesh can be fixated using a laparoscopic tacking device.

27. Typically mesh is fixated to either Cooper's ligament or the pubic bone, anteromedial and anterolateral.

28. After the mesh is secure, the peritoneal flap is closed with further tacks or a suture.
29. The 12 mm trocar site fascial defect is closed using a fascial closure device or under direct vision.
30. The pneumoperitoneum is released and the skin incisions are closed.

Chapter 36
Rives-Stoppa Ventral Hernia Repair

Justin Chamberlain

Overview

- Make midline laparotomy incision
- Perform adhesiolysis to free abdominal wall of all bowel and attachements
- Separate the anterior and posterior rectus sheaths to the level of the arcuate line
- Dissect the rectus abdominis off the posterior rectus sheath to the linea semilunaris
- Close the posterior rectus sheath
- Place mesh in the retrorectus space; can suture in place (attending dependent)
- Place JP drain in retrorectus space and close the anterior rectus sheath
- Excise any excess skin and close

Clinical Pearls

- Anterior rectus sheath is comprised of external oblique fascia plus anterior leaflet of the internal oblique fascia

J. Chamberlain (✉)
ProMedica Physicians General Surgery, Monroe, MI, USA
e-mail: Justin.Chamberlain@ProMedica.org

© Springer Nature Switzerland AG 2020　　　　　　　　217
E. Karamanos (ed.), *Common Surgeries Made Easy*,
https://doi.org/10.1007/978-3-030-41350-7_36

- Posterior rectus sheath is comprised of the transversalis fascia plus the posterior leaflet of the internal oblique fascia
- The posterior rectus sheath fuses with the anterior rectus sheath to run anterior to the rectus abdominis at the arcuate line
  - The intersection point of the arcuate line with the linea semilunaris is where Spigealian hernias occur
- The neurovascular bundle to the rectus abdominis runs between the rectus abdominis and the posterior rectus sheath

Patient Preparation

The patient should receive appropriate preoperative antibiotic prophylaxis aimed at decreasing the risk of superficial surgical site infection, usually a first generation cephalosporin. Pre-operative subcutaneous unfractionated heparin or low-dose low molecular weight heparin administration has been shown to decrease the risk of postoperative venous thromboembolism and does not increase the risk of significant intraoperative or postoperative bleeding and should be given. Prior to induction of anesthesia sequential compression devices are placed. After induction a Foley catheter is placed. The patient is positioned supine on the operating table with both arms fully abducted to allow the surgeon to stand as close to the abdomen as possible.

Anesthesia

General endotracheal anesthesia is necessary for this operation. Preoperative or postoperative epidural catheter placement may significantly improve pain management and decrease narcotic requirements in the post-operative period and should be considered. Communication with anesthesia throughout the surgery is essential to ensure complete paralysis during attempts at fascial advancement.

Skin Incision

The skin incision for each ventral hernia repair must be tailored to each patient's hernia morphology, but general principles may be followed. Palpation is used to mark the edge of the fascial defect bilaterally. The skin between the fascial edges is most often excised as part of the operation, however based on surgeon preference and proximity to underlying bowel the initial incision may be made in the midline directly over the hernia defect or along the edge of the defect at the fascial edge. In either case care must be taken to incise only skin and hernia sac and to avoid injuring underlying bowel or fascia.

Operative Steps

1. Prep and drape the abdomen into a sterile field. Ensure that the prep extends laterally widely in case lateral incisions must be made for relaxing incisions.
2. Incise the skin and hernia sac overlying the ventral hernia. Take care to avoid injuring the underlying bowel or fascia.
3. Using sharp Metzenbaum scissors lyse adhesions between the underlying bowel and hernia sac.
4. Once the hernia sac is freed from underlying adhesions excise the hernia sac and the skin overlying it using a sharp knife.
5. Starting on one side of the abdomen, grasp the fascial edge using several Kocher clamps and retract it medially and towards the ceiling. Using gentle pressure towards the table on the underlying bowel to create counter traction, sharply lyse adhesions between the bowel and the anterior abdominal wall moving laterally to the peri-colic gutter. A lap sponge may be used to gain traction on slippery bowel.
6. Repeat this process on the other side of the abdomen. Again, care must be taken to avoid injuring underlying bowel, but if it is injured it should be repaired immediately at the time of discovery.

7. Once the entire anterior abdominal wall is freed of adhesions attention is turned to developing the retro-rectus plane. Choose a location above the arcuate line and make a small incision at the junction of the anterior and posterior rectus fascia using Bovie (Fig. 36.1).

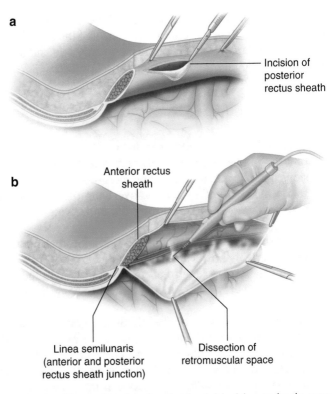

a — Incision of posterior rectus sheath

b Anterior rectus sheath

Linea semilunaris (anterior and posterior rectus sheath junction)

Dissection of retromuscular space

FIGURE 36.1 Illustration showing the fascial incision to begin separating the antior and posterior rectus sheaths. Typically the incision is made towards the posterior sheath to avoid wasting any of the anterior sheath. All usable width of the anterior sheath must be maintained to allow successful closure of the anterior fascia in the midline

8. Using a right angle clamp inserted into this space extend this incision cranially and caudally to separate the anterior and posterior fascia. The posterior rectus fascia stops at the arcuate line and this plane becomes continuous with the pre-peritoneal space there. Care must be taken at this location to maintain the integrity of the peritoneum which is much more fragile than the posterior fascia.

9. Grasp the anterior fascia using several Kocher clamps and retract it towards the ceiling. Grasp the posterior fascia using either Allis clamps, Lahey clamps, or Vulsellum clamps and retract it medially and posteriorly.

10. Use Bovie to sharply develop the retro-rectus plane immediately above the posterior fascia above the arcuate line or peritoneum below it. This plane is avascular and if bleeding is encountered it generally means the plane is off.

11. During the development of this plane several neurovascular bundles to the rectus muscle will be encountered. These should be preserved and lifted anteriorly along with the rectus muscle.

12. Develop this plane laterally until the semilunar line is encountered. Make sure to not incise the semilunar line.

13. Repeat this development of the retro-rectus plane on the other side of the abdomen.

14. Once the retro-rectus plane is developed bilaterally, grasp the anterior rectus fascia on both sides using Kocher clamps and advance them to the midline. If the fascia reaches the midline without undue tension, proceed with posterior fascial closure and retro rectus mesh placement. If not, additional maneuvers such as external oblique release or transversus abdominis release may be attempted to allow further fascial advancement. These releases are outside the scope of this chapter.

15. Close any tears in the posterior fascia above the arcuate line or peritoneum below the arcuate line using interrupted suture of 2–0 PDS. Ensure sponge and needle counts are correct prior to beginning posterior fascial closure.

16. Close the posterior rectus fascia above the arcuate line and the peritoneum below the arcuate line in a running fashion using a 2–0 PDS suture.

17. Using a sterile ruler to measure the length and width of the retro rectus plane.

18. Trim a large pore medium weight uncoated permanent mesh to fit the retro rectus space.

19. Place the trimmed mesh so it lies in the retro-rectus space without wrinkles or curled up edges.

20. Bring a 19 French round Jackson-Pratt drain through the abdominal wall remote to the midline abdominal incision and into the retro rectus space overlying the hernia mesh.

21. Close the anterior fascia in a running fashion using an 0 PDS suture beginning cranially and caudally with 2 separate suture lines and meeting in the middle. Care must be taken not to suture the drain in place during the fascial closure.

22. Close the Scarpa's fascia using interrupted 3–0 Vicryl sutures.

23. Ensure that all redundant skin and scar is trimmed from the skin edges.

24. Close skin using surgical staples or subcuticular sutures with 4–0 Vicryl or 4–0 Monocryl per surgeon's preference. Apply a sterile dressing of choice.

Chapter 37
Anterior Component Separation

Michael Sippel, Nicholas Robbins, and Amita Shah

Overview

- Make midline laparotomy
- Perform extensive adhesiolysis to free abdominal wall of all bowel and attachements
- Make lipocutaneous flaps anterior to anterior rectus sheath, extending 2 cm lateral to linea semilunaris
- Make small nic in external oblique fascia 1–2 cm lateral to linea semilunaris, and extend cranially and caudally
- Bluntly dissect external oblique muscle off the fascia
- Bring anterior rectus sheath together at midline
- Can perform an undelay or overlay mesh placement
- Place JP drains above the anterior rectus sheath

M. Sippel • N. Robbins
Department of Surgery, UT Health San Antonio,
San Antonio, TX, USA

A. Shah (✉)
Division of Plastic and Reconstructive Surgery, UT Health San
Antonio, San Antonio, TX, USA
e-mail: shahar@uthscsa.edu

© Springer Nature Switzerland AG 2020
E. Karamanos (ed.), *Common Surgeries Made Easy*,
https://doi.org/10.1007/978-3-030-41350-7_37

Clinical Pearls

- Anterior rectus sheath is comprised of external oblique fascia plus anterior leaflet of the internal oblique fascia
- Posterior rectus sheath is comprised of the transversalis fascia plus the posterior leaflet of the internal oblique fascia
- Flap necrosis is feared complication as perforators supplying blood flow can be disrupted

  - Can be performed minimally invasively with laparoscope, balloon dissector, and hook cautery

Patient Placement

Supine, with arms abducted. Consider a nasogastric tube. A Foley indicated due to operative time. Prep the patient with chlorhexidine from the nipples to the pubic symphysis.

Anesthesia

General Endotracheal. Consider an epidural catheter placement.

Operative Steps

1. Midline laparotomy incision, lysis of any adhesions, inspection of the abdominal wall for hernias or defects, removal of foreign bodies (tacks, suture, mesh, etc.), and identification of the fascia medial to the rectus abdominis should be completed as previously outlined.
2. Dissect the subcutaneous fat off the anterior rectus creating lipocutaneous flaps.

(a) Superior border: costal margin
(b) Inferior border: inguinal ligament
(c) Lateral border: approximately 1–2 cm lateral to linea semilunaris (this is where the external oblique is released),

3. Release the external oblique aponeurosis 1–2 cm lateral to linea semilunaris from just above the costal margin to just below the inguinal ligament (Fig. 37.1).
4. Assess if the linea alba can be reapproximated without tension. If the linea alba can be recreated without undue tension, then reapproximate the rectus midline. If this cannot be done without undue tension, consider a posterior component separation as well.
5. Once the abdomen is closed, attention to peak airway pressure, urine output, and blood pressure is important to ensure closure has not caused significant elevation in intra-abdominal pressure.
6. Onlay mesh placement: Place mesh over the closed midline repair and suture to the lateral cut edges of the external oblique.
7. Place drains (2–4) in a dependent position over the mesh.
8. Assess the skin flaps and remove any subscarpa fat which appears ischemic. Skin flaps can be sutured to the abdominal wall (reducing dead space).
9. Close the subcutaneous tissue in layers (3–0 Vicryl suture), and reapproximate the skin (4–0 Monocryl suture or staples). Consider removing redundant skin from the midline if present.

Disclaimers

"The views expressed are those of the [author(s)] [presenter(s)] and do not reflect the official views or policy of the Department of Defense or its Components"

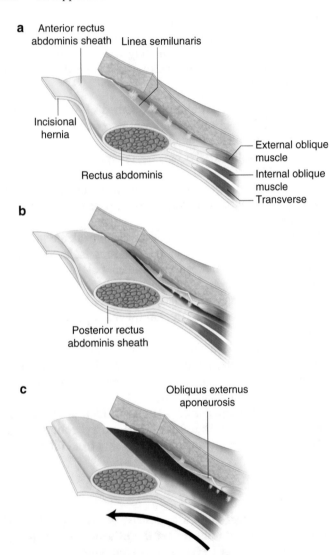

FIGURE 37.1 During anterior component separation, the aponeurosis of the external oblique is divided, allowing en - block advancement of the rectus abdominis/internal oblique/transversus abdominis towards the midline in order to reconstruct the midline

Chapter 38
Posterior Component Separation

Michael Sippel, Nicholas Robbins, and Amita Shah

Overview

- Make midline laparotomy
- Perform extensive adhesiolysis to free abdominal wall of all bowel and attachments
- Separate the anterior and posterior rectus sheaths to the level of the arcuate line
- Dissect the rectus abdominis off the posterior rectus sheath to the linea semilunaris
- Incise posterior rectus sheath 0.5 cm medial to linea semilunaris
- Dissect rectus abdominis from posterior rectus sheath
- Perform intramuscular dissection by dividing internal oblique muscle
- If performing transversus abdominis release, dissect transversus abdominis off transversalis fascia from costal margin to myopectineal orifice and lateral to psoas muscles

M. Sippel · N. Robbins
Department of Surgery, UT Health San Antonio, San Antonio, TX, USA

A. Shah (✉)
Division of Plastic and Reconstructive Surgery, UT Health San Antonio, San Antonio, TX, USA
e-mail: shahar@uthscsa.edu

© Springer Nature Switzerland AG 2020
E. Karamanos (ed.), *Common Surgeries Made Easy*,
https://doi.org/10.1007/978-3-030-41350-7_38

- Perform underlay or retrorectus mesh placement, and close posterior rectus sheath
- Close anterior rectus sheath
- JP drain placement above anterior rectus sheath

Clinical Pearls

- Anterior rectus sheath is comprised of external oblique fascia plus anterior leaflet of the internal oblique fascia
- Posterior rectus sheath is comprised of the transversalis fascia plus the posterior leaflet of the internal oblique fascia
- Inferior and superior epigastric vessels travel between rectus abdominis and posterior rectus sheath
- PCS can be combined with transversus abdominis release surgery to gain more laxity for tension-free closure
- PCS plus TARS has 5% hernia recurrence rate at 2 years, and avoids the creation of large lipocutaneous flaps at risk of flap necrosis

Patient Placement

Supine, with arms abducted. Consider a nasogastric tube. A Foley indicated due to operative time. Prep the patient with chlorhexidine prep from the nipples to the pubic symphysis.

Anesthesia

General Endotracheal. Consider an epidural catheter placement.

Operative Steps

1. A midline laparotomy incision is made. Of note, the incision should not be carried past the pubis on morbidly obese patients due to skin care issues.

2. Carry the dissection midline through the subcutaneous tissue and identify the linea alba.
3. Enter the abdominal cavity in the usual fashion.
4. Perform any necessary lysis of adhesions and define the fascial edges of the rectus abdominis.
5. Remove any foreign material (tacks, suture, mesh).
6. Place a moist sterile towel over the viscera for protection during the remainder of the operation.
7. With the electrocautery device, make an incision in the posterior rectus sheath 0.5 cm from the medial border (just medial to the linea alba). Carry this incision cranial and caudal, spanning the entire length of the rectus abdominis muscle.
8. With the electrocautery device and the use of blunt dissection, continue this plane lateral to the linea semilunaris. Care must be taken to preserve the inferior epigastric vessels, which should remain within the muscle, not the posterior sheath.
9. Extend this plane superiorly to the retroxiphoid/retrosternal space, and inferiorly to the space of Retzius. This allows for exposure of the midline symphysis pubis and the Cooper's ligaments bilaterally.
10. If the dissection of the retrorectus space is insufficient to allow adequate component advancement, then retrorectus dissection lateral to linea semilunaris can be accomplished by an intramuscular dissection (dividing internal oblique), dissection within the preperitoneal plane, or a transversus abdominis release.
11. Incise the posterior sheath using an electrocautery device 0.5 cm medial to the linea semilunaris to expose the transversus abdominus muscle. The muscle belly is well defined in the superior aspect of the abdominal wall, begin dissection here.
12. Transect the transversus abdominus muscle with an electrocautery device. Keep in mind the transversalis fascia and the peritoneum are deep here (Fig. 38.1).
13. Retract the transversus abdominus anteriorly and develop the retromuscular plane bluntly. Superior: beyond the costal margin to the diaphragm; inferior: to the myopectineal orifice; lateral: psoas muscle.

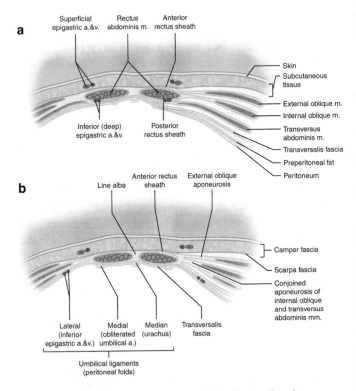

FIGURE 38.1 Anatomy of the anterior abdominal wall and transverse abdominis release

14. Complete the Transversus Abdominus Release (TAR) of the contralateral side in the same fashion.
15. Reapproximate the posterior rectus sheath in the midline using Vicryl sutures (2–0). Any holes created during dissection or previous operations must be closed.
16. Orient the mesh into a diamond configuration and anchor it inferiorly, just superior to the pubic ramus or bilaterally into Cooper's ligament. The mesh can be positioned in the space of Retzius to address any lower midline defects, positioned to cover the myopectineal orifice(s) in the setting of concurrent inguinal or femoral hernias, or beyond

the costal margin for any superior midline defects. The mesh is then anchored with transfacial stitches (3–0 PDS suture) adjacent to the xiphoid process.

17. Place Kocher clamps on the medial edge of the rectus muscle, pull toward the midline, and place full thickness transfascial sutures (3–0 PDS suture) to secure the mesh in 3 cardinal points as a sublay in the retromuscular space. This allows for primary fascial closure over the mesh and reduces midline tension. Perform the contralateral side in the same fashion.

18. Once the mesh has been circumferentially secured, place drains (2–4) superficial to the mesh in the dependent sites of the repair. Reapproximate the anterior rectus sheath in the midline, recreating the linea alba. Attention to peak airway pressure, urine output, and blood pressure is important here to ensure closure has not caused significant elevation in intra-abdominal pressure.

19. Close the subcutaneous tissue in layers (3–0 Vicryl suture), and close the skin (4–0 Monocryl suture or staples).

Disclaimers

"The views expressed are those of the [author(s)] [presenter(s)] and do not reflect the official views or policy of the Department of Defense or its Components"

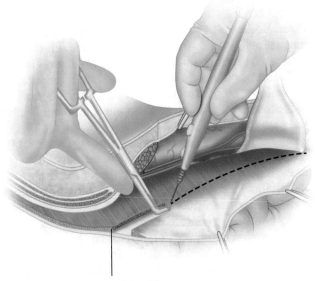

Transversus abdominis
release (TAR)

Part IX
Breast

Chapter 39
Simple Mastectomy

Kelly Rosso

Overview

- Make elliptical incision to include NAC and down to subcutaneous fat
- Using electrocautery, dissect plane between breast tissue and subcutaneous fat

  - This plan is avascular, and should not bleed

- Dissection should be carried to clavicle superiorly, latissimus dorsi laterally, sternum medially, and inferior mammary fold inferiorly
- Remove specimen en bloc including pectoralis major fascia

Clinical Pearls

- BiRADs Classification

  - 0: nondiagnostic, repeat mammogram
  - 1: negative, routine screening
  - 2: benign findings, routine screening

K. Rosso (✉)
Department of Surgical Oncology, Banner MD Anderson Cancer Center, Gilbert, AZ, USA

© Springer Nature Switzerland AG 2020
E. Karamanos (ed.), *Common Surgeries Made Easy*,
https://doi.org/10.1007/978-3-030-41350-7_39

235

- 3: likely benign, repeat in 6 months
- 4: suspicious abnormality, diagnostic mammogram and biopsy warranted
- 5: suggestive of malignancy, biopsy warranted
- 6: known malignancy

- Nipple sparing mastectomy preserves the nipple areolar complex and is oncologically safe for risk reduction and cancer treatment in the appropriate patient
- Must ensure that mastectomy flap is not too thin as this will lead to flap necrosis, nor that it is too thick, thus leaving behind breast tissue and increasing risk of recurrence
- Hormonal therapy and trastuzumab are contraindicated in pregnancy
- Chemotherapy is ok to use in 2nd and 3rd trimesters

Patient Placement

The patient is positioned supine with both arms gently abducted and secured to arm boards. The ipsilateral arm may be prepped circumferentially and included in the field if a sentinel lymph node or an axillary lymph node dissection is planned.

Anesthesia

General endotracheal anesthesia is standard. Pre-induction paravertebral or intercostal nerve blocks may decrease postoperative opioid use and improve overall pain control.

Landmarks and Skin Incision

The mastectomy flaps are created superiorly to the clavicle, medially to the sternum, inferiorly to the rectus abdominis fascia, and laterally to the latissimus dorsi muscle. The incision for a total mastectomy without reconstruction is an

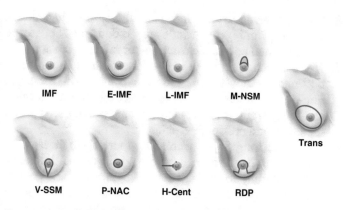

IMF   **E-IMF**   **L-IMF**   **M-NSM**

Trans

V-SSM   **P-NAC**   **H-Cent**   **RDP**

FIGURE 39.1 Different mastectomy skin incisions

ellipse shaped incision that can be closed primarily with minimal redundant skin under minimal tension. The incision used for a skin sparing mastectomy is made just outside the boundary of the nipple areolar complex to ensure preservation of the skin envelope for reconstruction. An incision at the inframammary fold may be utilized with a nipple sparing mastectomy technique. The skin and nipple sparing techniques require a good light source and a good assistant. The operative steps below will describe a total mastectomy without reconstruction (Fig. 39.1).

Operative Steps

1. Mark the planned resection boundaries with a skin marker: The clavicle superiorly, the lateral border of the sternum medially, the rectus abdominis fascia inferiorly and the latissimus dorsi muscle laterally. If a sentinel lymph node biopsy is planned, perform an intraoperative lymphatic mapping by injection of blue dye and radiolabeled colloid (both the sentinel lymph node dissection and the axillary lymph node dissections were described elsewhere).

2. Use a 15 blade scalpel and make the ellipse shaped skin incision, planning to include any redundant skin in the resection and ensure a closure under minimal tension.

3. Use an electrocautery device, to dissect through the plane between the breast tissue and the subcutaneous tissue. The non-dominant hand is used to retract the breast inferiorly and away from your dissection plane, putting tension on the plane and making it visible.

4. The mastectomy flaps are created superiorly to the clavicle, medially to the sternum, inferiorly to the rectus abdominis fascia, laterally to the latissimus dorsi muscle and continued to include the tail of Spence. Care is taken to preserve the medial perforating vessels. Maintaining impeccable dissection in the correct plane preserves blood supply to the flap and helps prevent ischemia or necrosis.

5. Continue the dissection to the chest wall and remove the breast en bloc to include the pectoralis major fascia. Mark the breast with orienting sutures and submit to pathology.

6. Irrigate the axilla with warm saline and achieve hemostasis. Place a single 15 round Blake drain in the wound, brought out through a separate stab incision, and secured to the skin with a 2–0 Nylon suture.

7. Close the wound using a 3–0 Vicryl suture in an interrupted deep dermal fashion, followed by a running subcuticular 4–0 Monocryl suture.

Chapter 40
Lumpectomy and Sentinel Lymph Node Biopsy

Kelly Rosso

Overview

- Preoperatively, patient sent to IR for Lymophoscintigraphy and wire localization
- Isofluran blue dye is infiltrated into subdermal space around tumor before incision
- Make incision along border of areola, inframammary fold, or Langer's line depending on tumor location
- Dissect down towards mass, delivering wire into the surgical wound
- Excise mass and wire
- Using probe, find area of highest reactivity, and make incision in axilla
- Dissect down to and through clavipectoral fascia
- Using combination of probe and visualization, find hot, blue node and measure radioactivity
- Remove all nodes that reach 10% threshold

K. Rosso (✉)
Department of Surgical Oncology, Banner MD Anderson Cancer Center, Gilbert, AZ, USA

© Springer Nature Switzerland AG 2020
E. Karamanos (ed.), *Common Surgeries Made Easy*,
https://doi.org/10.1007/978-3-030-41350-7_40

239

Clinical Pearls

- Contraindications to Breast Conservation Therapy

    - Two or more primary tumors
    - 1st or 2nd trimester pregnancy
    - Persistent positive margins
    - Prior radiation to chest
    - Multicentric Disease
    - Small breast/Large mass
    - Scleroderma

- BiRADs Classification

    - 0: nondiagnostic, repeat mammogram
    - 1: negative, routine screening
    - 2: benign findings, routine screening
    - 3: likely benign, repeat in 6 months
    - 4: suspicious abnormality, diagnostic mammogram and biopsy warranted
    - 5: suggestive of malignancy, biopsy warranted
    - 6: known malignancy

- Hormonal therapy and trastuzumab are contraindicated in pregnancy
- Dye is teratogenic, only use radiotracer in pregnancy
- Chemotherapy is ok to use in 2nd and 3rd trimesters

Patient Placement

The patient is positioned supine with both arms gently abducted and secured to arm boards. If there is a possibility for a completion axillary lymph node dissection at the time of surgery (for instance, a positive sentinel lymph node is identified by immediate frozen assessment for those patients who have received neoadjuvant chemotherapy), the ipsilateral arm may be prepped circumferentially and included in the field. Adducting the arm with a bent elbow during completion axillary lymph node dissection allows for easier access to level II nodes, posterior to the pectoralis minor muscle.

Anesthesia

General endotracheal anesthesia is standard. 0.25% Marcaine may be infiltrated into the surgical site for analgesia. If using Isosulfan blue for intraoperative lymphatic mapping, blue dye prophylaxis with Famotidine 20 mg, Benadryl 50 mg, and Decadron 4 mg is given intravenously around the time of induction.

Landmarks and Skin Incision

The breast incision typically depends on where the wire or seed is placed to localize the tumor. The incision can be made at the areolar border or near the inframammary fold for cosmetic purposes. An incision along Langer's lines is also adequate. Planning for the sentinel lymph node biopsy incision must consider the possibility of conversion to axillary lymph node dissection. Identify and mark the lateral borders of the pectoralis major muscle and the latissimus dorsi muscle. The sentinel lymph node biopsy incision is made in a skin fold, inferior to the inferior most hair follicles in the axilla.

Operative Steps

Prior to prepping, inject Isosulfan blue dye in the peritumoral location or in the retroareolar space. Technetium sulfur colloid is injected into the subareolar region. After injection of blue dye, the breast is massaged gently for 5 minutes. Prep the operative field using chlorhexidine.

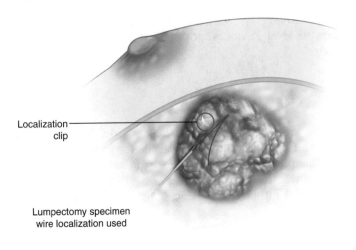

Localization clip

Lumpectomy specimen wire localization used

FIGURE 40.1 Partial mastectomy with the aid of wire localization

Lumpectomy
1. Identify the region of the breast that contains the wire (or radioactive seed) localized mass by palpation and assessment of the preoperative images.
1. Using a 15 blade, make an incision along Langer's lines, along the areolar border or at the inframammary fold.
2. Use electrocautery to create lumpectomy flaps superiorly, inferiorly, medially, and laterally surrounding the mass and needle tip.
3. Remove the wire tip and deliver the wire into the incision using hemostats. Do not displace the wire with this step.
4. Deepen the circumferential margins around the mass.
5. Grasp the lumpectomy specimen gently, deliver through the incision with an Allis clamp and excise the posterior border to include pectoralis fascia if the tumor is posterior or abutting the muscle (Fig. 40.1).
6. Mark the lumpectomy specimen with a short stitch at the superior margin, a long stitch at the lateral margin, and ink at the posterior margin. Immediate specimen radiograph should demonstrate the intact wire (or seed), biopsy clip and associated mass.

7. Irrigate with warm saline, suction dry, obtain hemostasis with electrocautery and place metallic clips to facilitate future identification of the operative cavity. Close with interrupted a 3–0 monocryl suture to reapproximate the deep tissues and dermis, followed by a 4–0 monocryl suture running subcuticular suture.

Sentinel Lymph Node biopsy

1. Use the probe to identify the region of strongest radioactive signal, and make an incision using a 15-blade scalpel over this area. Deepen through the subcutaneous tissue and open the clavipectoral fascia.
2. Identify all blue lymph nodes and/or those with radio uptake while clipping afferent lymphatics and dissecting free of the surrounding tissue to excise. Preserve the intercostal nerves if possible.
3. Once the axilla is surveyed and counts are <10% of the highest sentinel lymph node, the nodal sampling is complete. Gently palpate to identify any abnormal nodes that may not have been identified by intraoperative lymphatic mapping and submit those nodes as "non-sentinel lymph nodes" if found.
4. Irrigate the cavity, suction dry, obtain hemostasis and close the axilla in three layers, that includes re-approximation of the clavipectoral fascia, deep dermal skin and subcuticular layer.

Chapter 41
Axillary Lymph Node Dissection

Kelly Rosso

Overview

- Curvilinear incision made at posterior aspect of pectoralis major
- Dissect down to clavipectoral fascia and open to enter axilla
- Identify latissimus dorsi and dissect up to axillary vein
- Identify thoracodorsal bundle and long thoracic nerve and ensure to protect during dissection
- Excise all lymphatic tissue containing level I nodes
- Identify pectoralis minor muscle and excise all level II nodes posterior to muscle

Clinical Pearls

- Boundaries of Axilla

  - Superior: Axillary Vein
  - Medial: Pectoralis major
  - Posterior: Latissimus dorsi
  - Anterior: Clavipectoral fascia

K. Rosso (✉)
Department of Surgical Oncology, Banner MD Anderson Cancer Center, Gilbert, AZ, USA

© Springer Nature Switzerland AG 2020
E. Karamanos (ed.), *Common Surgeries Made Easy*,
https://doi.org/10.1007/978-3-030-41350-7_41

245

- Dissection superior to axillary vein can result in brachial plexus injury and increased lymphedema risk
- Long thoracic nerve innervates serratus anterior
  - Injury results in winged scapula
- Thoracodorsal nerve innervates lattisimus dorsi
  - Injury results in weakness in adduction >90 degrees
- Axillary Lymph Node Levels
  - I: lateral to pectoralis minor

    included in ax dissection
  - II: behind pectoralis minor

    included in ax dissection
  - III: medial to pectoralis minor
- Rotor's Nodes: between pectoralis major and minor muscles
- Stewart Treves Syndrome
  - Lymphangiosarcoma secondary to chronic lymphedema following ax dissection
  - Will present with dark purple nodular lesions on arm 5–10 years after surgery

Patient Placement

The patient is positioned supine with both arms gently abducted and secured to arm boards. The ipsilateral arm may be prepped circumferentially and included in the field. Adducting the arm with a bent elbow during completion axillary lymph node dissection allows for easier access to level II nodes, posterior to the pectoralis minor muscle.

Anesthesia

General endotracheal anesthesia is standard. Ensure that no paralytic agents are used as the thoracodorsal neurovascular bundle and long thoracic nerve must be identified. Paravertebral or intercostal nerve blocks may decrease post-operative opioid use and improve overall pain control.

Landmarks and Skin Incision

Identify and mark the lateral borders of the pectoralis major muscle and the latissimus dorsi muscle. A curvilinear or "lazy S" incision is made starting posterior to the lateral border of the pectoralis major muscle and ending just anterior to the lateral border of the latissimus dorsi muscle.

Operative Steps

1. After prepping with chlorhexidine and identifying landmarks described above. Make a curvilinear or "lazy S" incision in the axillary skin with a 15 blade and deepen into the subcutaneous tissue with an electrocautery device.
2. Identify the pectoralis major muscle anteromedially. At the lateral border of the pectoralis major muscle, open the clavipectoral fascia.
3. Identify the latissimus dorsi muscle in the posterolateral aspect of the dissection and expose the muscle along its length to the level of the axillary vein.
4. Identify and preserve the thoracodorsal nerve bundle coursing along the anterior aspect of the muscle and follow cephalad to its insertion in the axillary vein.

5. Identify and preserve the long thoracic nerve as it courses along the chest wall, lateral to the serratus anterior muscle.

6. All intervening lymphatic tissue is excised en bloc and sent to pathology for permanent evaluation (Fig. 41.1).

7. Identify the pectoralis minor muscle and excise additional level II axillary lymph nodes posterior to it.

8. Palpate for level III disease, medial to the pectoralis minor muscle. Occasionally, the pectoralis minor muscle must be taken down at its insertion to access and adequately dissect level III nodes.

9. Irrigate the axilla with warm saline and achieve hemostasis. Place a single 15 round Blake drain in the wound, brought out through a separate stab incision, and secured to the skin with a 2–0 Nylon suture.

10. Close the wound using a 3–0 Vicryl suture in an interrupted deep dermal fashion, followed by a running subcuticular 4.0 Monocryl suture.

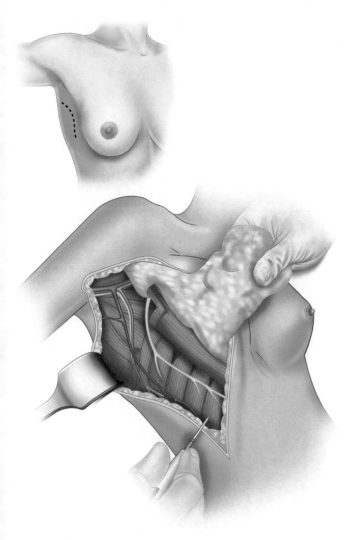

FIGURE 41.1 Incision for axillary lymphadenectomy and important axillary structures that need to be preserved

Part X
Endocrine

Chapter 42
Thyroidectomy

Sophie Dream

Overview

- Transverse incision two fingerbreadths above sternal notch
- Divide platysma and raise subplatysmal flaps
- Divide strap muscles midline and retract laterally
- Expose thyroid gland and dissect sternothyroid muscle off thyroid
- Dissect upper pole, then open the space of Reeves to define medial aspect of upper pole
- Identify and ligate superior thyroid vessels
- Identify and ligate middle thyroid vein
- Identify and protect the recurrent laryngeal nerve, and parathyroid glands
- Dissect to isthmus, identifying and ligating terminal branches of inferior thyroid artery and vein
- If performing total thyroidectomy, complete above steps on contralateral side
- If performing hemithyroidectomy, dissect through the thyroid isthmus with energy device
- Dissect thyroid off trachea

S. Dream (✉)
Division of Surgical Oncology, University of Alabama,
Birmingham, AL, USA

© Springer Nature Switzerland AG 2020
E. Karamanos (ed.), *Common Surgeries Made Easy*,
https://doi.org/10.1007/978-3-030-41350-7_42

Clinical Pearls

- Preop workup of thyroid nodule includes neck ultrasound, TFT's, FNA biopsy
- Ensure that hyperthyroidism is adequately controlled prior to surgery as this may increase perioperative risks
- Recurrent laryngeal nerve will run in tracheoesophageal groove and courses behind the inferior thryroid artery → innervates all intrinsic muscles of larynx except for crico-thyroid muscle

    - Unilateral injury to RLN will result in horseness
    - Bilateral injury can result in vocal cord paralysis and will lie in paramedian position, unable to open during inspiration → can necessitate tracheostomy

- External Branch of the superior laryngeal nerve courses posterior to internal carotid artery → innervates the crico-thyroid muscle

    - Injury results in decreased pitch

- Nerve monitoring

    - Communication with anesthesia team to avoid muscle relaxation.
    - Endotracheal intubation with electrode placed under direct laryngoscopy to ensure electrode are in contact with the true vocal cords.
    - Placement of ground wires under skin of the sternum or shoulder.
    - After incision, test stimulator on the sternocleidomastoid muscle to confirm muscle twitching.
    - Divide median raphe and elevate the sternothyroid muscle off the sternohyoid muscle.
    - Continue in this place laterally until the carotid artery is reached.
    - Stimulate the vagus nerve here at the beginning of the operation.

- Once recurrent laryngeal nerve is identified, stimulate to confirm and map out the course.
- Prior to closure, stimulate the recurrent nerve and the vagus nerve

- Lymph Node Stations
  - I: submandibular, submandibular
  - II: superior jugular
  - III: middle jugular
  - IV: inferior jugular
  - V: posterior triangle
  - VI: central neck, anterior compartment

Positioning

Supine with arms tucked. A shoulder roll may help with neck extension. No need for a foley or preoperative antibiotics. Mechanical DVT prophylaxis. Prep the neck and upper chest.

Anesthesia

General anesthesia with endotracheal intubation is safe and most commonly used.

One may employ regional anesthesia using a cervical block in select patients.

Operative Steps

1. Make a transverse incision in a skin crease two finger-breadths above the sternal notch, below the cricoid cartilage.
2. Divide the subcutaneous tissues and the platysma.
3. Raise the subplatysmal flaps inferiorly to the sternal notch, superiorly to the thyroid cartilage. The plane of dis-

section will be superficial to the anterior jugular veins, which may be ligated to facilitate the dissection.

4. Suture the subplatysmal flaps for retraction, do not include the dermis.
5. Divide the sternohyoid and sternothyroid strap muscles in the midline and retract laterally.
6. Expose the thyroid gland and mobilize the thyroid lobe from the areolar tissue, dissecting the sternothyroid muscle off the thyroid gland.
7. Dissect the upper thyroid pole free from the surrounding connective tissue.
8. Bluntly open the cricothyroid space of Reeves (the avascular plane between the upper pole and the cricothyroid muscle) and define the medial aspect of the upper pole of the thyroid. This aids in identification of the external laryngeal nerve.
9. Retract the thyroid inferomedial.
10. Identify and ligate the superior vessels with clips.
11. Retract the lobe medially.
12. Identify and ligate the middle thyroid vein.
13. Identify and dissect out the recurrent laryngeal nerve, it is often located medial to the Tubercle of Zuckerkandl (the posterolateral aspect of the thyroid gland which is present in 80% of cases)(Fig. 42.1).
14. Identify and preserve the parathyroid glands.
15. Dissect to the isthmus along the thyroid capsule, taking the terminal branches of the inferior thyroid artery and vein.
16. Repeat steps 6–15 for the contralateral lobe.
17. Dissect the thyroid free of any attachments to the trachea at the ligament of Berry, with care to preserve the recurrent laryngeal nerve.
18. Mark the specimen for orientation.
19. Irrigate and achieve hemostasis.
20. Reapproximate the strap muscles with simple interrupted absorbable sutures.
21. Reapproximate the platysma with simple interrupted absorbable sutures.
22. Close the skin with deep dermal interrupted sutures and skin glue.

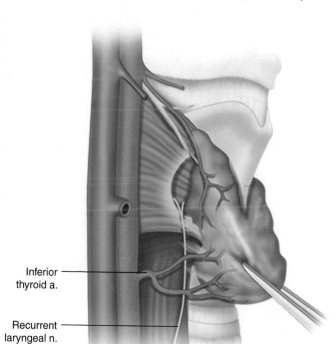

Inferior
thyroid a.

Recurrent
laryngeal n.

FIGURE 42.1 Anatomic relationships of artery and nerve in thyroid lobecotmy

Chapter 43
Thyroid Lobectomy

Sophie Dream

Positioning

Supine with arms tucked. A shoulder roll may help with neck extension. No need for a foley or preoperative antibiotics. Mechanical DVT prophylaxis. Prep the neck and upper chest.

Anesthesia

General anesthesia with endotracheal intubation is safe and most commonly used.

One may employ regional anesthesia using a cervical block in select patients.

Operative Steps

1. Perform a transverse incision in a skin crease two finger-breadths above the sternal notch, below the cricoid cartilage.
2. Divide the subcutaneous tissues and platysma.

S. Dream (✉)
Division of Surgical Oncology, University of Alabama, Birmingham, AL, USA

© Springer Nature Switzerland AG 2020
E. Karamanos (ed.), *Common Surgeries Made Easy*,
https://doi.org/10.1007/978-3-030-41350-7_43

3. Raise the subplatysmal flaps inferiorly to the sternal notch, superiorly to the thyroid cartilage. The plane of dissection will be superficial to the anterior jugular veins, which may be ligated to facilitate dissection.
4. Suture the subplatysmal flaps for retraction, do not include dermis.
5. Divide the sternohyoid and sternothyroid strap muscles in the midline and retract laterally.
6. Expose the thyroid gland and mobilize the thyroid lobe from any areolar tissue, dissecting the sternothyroid muscle off the thyroid gland.
7. Dissect the upper thyroid pole free from the surrounding connective tissue.
8. Bluntly open the cricothyroid space of Reeves and define the medial aspect of the upper pole of the thyroid.
9. Retract the thyroid inferomedial.
10. Identify and ligate the superior vessels.
11. Retract the lobe medially.
12. Identify and ligate the middle thyroid vein.
13. Identify and dissect out the recurrent laryngeal nerve.
14. Identify and preserve the parathyroid glands.
15. Retract the thyroid medially.
16. Dissect the lower pole along the thyroid capsule, taking the terminal branches of the inferior thyroid artery and vein.
17. Dissect the thyroid free of any attachments to the trachea at the ligament of Berry, with care to preserve the recurrent laryngeal nerve.
18. Dissect to the isthmus.
19. Clamp the thyroid and ligate.
20. Mark the specimen for orientation.
21. Irrigate and achieve hemostasis.
22. Reapproximate the strap muscles with simple interrupted absorbable sutures.
23. Reapproximate the platysma with simple interrupted absorbable sutures.
24. Close the skin with deep dermal interrupted sutures and skin glue.

Chapter 44
Parathyroidectomy

Sophie Dream

Overview

- Draw preop PTH
- Transverse incision two fingerbreadths above sternal notch
- Divide platysma and raise subplatysmal flaps
- Divide strap muscles midline and retract laterally
- Dissect thyroid from areolar tissue and retract anteriomedially
- Retract carotid sheath laterally
- Identify and trace recurrent laryngeal nerve to intersection with inferior thyroid artery to identify the superior and inferior parathyroid glands
- Identify the parathyroid adenoma, and clamp and ligate the pedicle
- If performing 4 gland exploration or 3.5 gland excision, explore contralateral side and clamp and ligate pedicles to each parathyroid
- Draw intraop PTH 10 minutes after adenoma or 3.5 gland excision performed
- If >50% drop from baseline, ok to close; if <50% drop, explore for ectopic adenoma or supernumerary gland

S. Dream (✉)
Division of Surgical Oncology, University of Alabama,
Birmingham, AL, USA

© Springer Nature Switzerland AG 2020
E. Karamanos (ed.), *Common Surgeries Made Easy*,
https://doi.org/10.1007/978-3-030-41350-7_44

Clinical Pearls

- Preop workup includes mulitple Ca levels, PTH, neck ultrasound vs. sestamibi scan, 24 hour urine Ca,
- Ectopic gland locations (Fig. 44.1)

    – Thymus gland (most common location)
    – Within carotid sheath
    – Tracheoesophageal groove
    – Within thyroid gland
    – If unable to find, and patient returns to OR at later date, most common location is in it's normal anatomic position

- Indications for surgery in asymptomatic patient

    – Ca >13
    – Cr clearance >30%
    – bone density t-score < −2.5
    – Urine Ca >400

- Minimally invasive vs. 4 gland exploration is controversial topic, and is attending dependent
- Postop hypocalcemia due to bone hunger (nl PTH, decreased HCO_3), or aparathyroidism (decreased PTH, nl HCO_3)

Positioning

Supine with arms tucked, shoulder roll the scapulae for neck extension. No need for a foley or preoperative antibiotics. Mechanical DVT prophylaxis. Prep the neck and the upper chest.

Anesthesia

General anesthesia with endotracheal intubation is safe and most commonly performed.

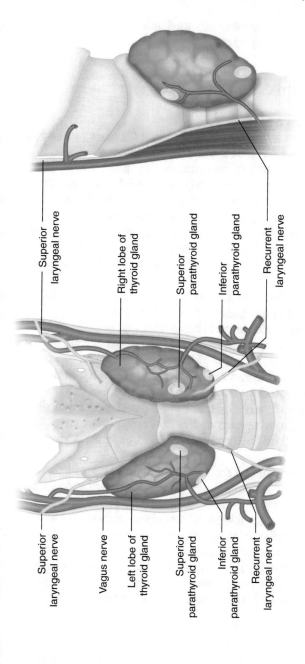

FIGURE 44.1 Anatomic location of parathyroids

One may employ regional anesthesia using a cervical block in select patients.

Operative Steps

1. Draw a baseline PTH.
2. Make a horizontal incision in a Langer's line two finger-breadths above the sternal notch.
3. Divide the subcutaneous tissues and platysma.
4. Raise subplatysmal flaps superficial to the anterior jugular veins, extend the flaps inferiorly to the sternal notch and superiorly to the thyroid cartilage.
5. Divide the sternohyoid and sternothyroid strap muscles in the midline, at the median raphe, and retract laterally.
6. Dissect the thyroid from the surrounding loose areolar tissue.
7. Mobilize and retract the thyroid anteromedially, may need to ligate the middle thyroid vein.
8. Retract the carotid sheath laterally.
9. Dissect along the medial aspect of the carotid artery.
10. Identify the point of intersection of the recurrent laryngeal nerve and the inferior thyroid artery, both superior and inferior glands will be within 1 cm of this point.
11. Identify any abnormal parathyroid gland and dissect it out from the surrounding tissue. An abnormal parathyroid gland will be firm, ballotable, larger than normal, darker in color.
12. Clamp and tie the pedicle of the parathyroid gland.
13. Survey the remaining glands for hyperplasia or double adenoma.
14. Excise any additional abnormal glands. In the case of hyperplastic glands, remove a portion of a lower gland prior to excising additional glands to ensure the remnant's viability. If the remnant does not appear viable, the contralateral lower gland may be used to fashion a remnant.
15. Draw a PTH at 10 minutes post-excision.

16. If the PTH does not drop by >50% of baseline level after 10 minutes, evaluate for an ectopic or supernumerary glands (see below), remove any additional glands until the PTH drops appropriately.
17. Irrigate and achieve hemostasis.
18. Reapproximate the strap muscles using interrupted, simple, absorbable sutures.
19. Reapproximate the platysma using interrupted, simple, absorbable sutures.
20. Close the skin with interrupted, simple, absorbable sutures in deep dermis and skin glue.

Part XI
Skin

Chapter 45
Split Thickness Skin Graft (STSG)

Claire Gerall, Jaclyn Yracheta, Michael Sippel, Nicholas Robbins, and Amita Shah

Overview

- Debride wound bed, measuring length, width, depth
- Identify donor site, select dermatome with correct width, and set correct depth
- Hold donor site taut, apply mineral oil
- Start dermatome and contact skin holding 45° angle with firm pressure
- When enough skin has been harvested, lift dermatome off skin
- Place STSG in saline and dress the donor site with epinephrine soaked gauze
- Mesh the STSG to desired ratio, then place and secure dermal side up on the wound bed
- Bolster vs. VAC the STSG, and dress the donor site

C. Gerall · J. Yracheta · M. Sippel · N. Robbins
Department of Surgery, UT Health San Antonio,
San Antonio, TX, USA

A. Shah (✉)
Division of Plastic and Reconstructive Surgery, UT Health San Antonio, San Antonio, TX, USA
e-mail: shahar@uthscsa.edu

© Springer Nature Switzerland AG 2020
E. Karamanos (ed.), *Common Surgeries Made Easy*,
https://doi.org/10.1007/978-3-030-41350-7_45

Clinical Pearls

- Stages of STSG survival
    - Imbibition (nutrients delivered by osmosis)
    - Inosculation (cut ends of vessels from STSG form connections to wound bed)
    - Angiogenesis
- Cosmetic areas should not use meshed STSG, pie crust graft to prevent seroma build-up
- Cannot graft over exposed joints or bone, use integra and then graft over integra in 3 weeks
- Possible iatrogenic causes of graft failure include
    - Seroma or hematoma formation
    - Infection at the recipient site
    - Failure to place the graft dermal side down
- Possible patient specific causes of graft failure include:
    - Obesity
    - Diabetes mellitus
    - Peripheral vascular disease

Patient Placement

Placement depends on the location of the wound. The patient is placed with the wound and the donor site accessible. The wound as well as the donor site (most commonly the anterior thigh or lower abdomen) are prepped and draped in the usual sterile manner. If possible, choose the donor site to be in an area that is easily hidden by clothing and that the patient will not be sitting or lying upon.

Anesthesia

General Endotracheal.

Operative Steps

1. Assess the open wound and debride any non-granulating tissue, ensuring there is no necrotic tissue or sign of infection. In wounds that have previously been infected, quantitative cultures of the operative area with bacterial loads less than 10^5 are recommended prior to skin grafting.
2. Measure the length, width, and depth of the wound to determine the size of the donor site.
3. Identify the donor site. Using a marking pen, mark the wound measurements at the donor site to ensure adequate donor tissue for wound coverage.
4. Apply sterile mineral oil to the donor site and to the dermatome.
5. Select a dermatome with the correct width and depth (0.2–0.4 mm) to harvest the donor skin.
6. Prepare to harvest the skin graft by applying tension on the distal and proximal areas of the skin graft to achieve a flat and taut donor site. In patients with loose skin or uneven contour, Tumescent solution consisting of 1 litre of lactated ringer's solution with 1–2 mg/L of epinephrine can be injected just under the skin using a 25 gauge spinal needle.
7. Turn on the dermatome prior to skin contact, hold the dermatome at a 45° angle and press against the skin with gentle, but firm, constant pressure. Slowly move down the donor site until you have harvested the appropriately sized graft. Remove the dermatome with the power still on to free the STSG from the donor site (Fig. 45.1).
8. Hold pressure at the donor site until hemostasis is achieved, then dress with xeroform, another non-adherent dressing, kerlix, and an ace wrap.
9. Wash the donor skin with saline and gently spread to avoid curled edges. The skin graft is then meshed at 1.5:1, sometimes 3:1 for larger defects. If one is unable to mesh or the donor skin is large, the skin may be prepared for grafting using a pie-crusting technique.

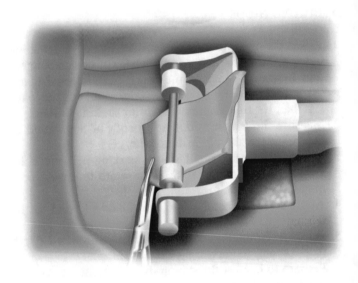

FIGURE 45.1 Harvesting of a split thickness skin graft

    (a) If a plastic carrier is being used, place the skin skin dermal side up on the carrier and spread the skin out. If a mesher with no carrier is being used, place the skin dermal side down.

    (b) Pass the carrier through the mesher, ensuring the graft stays on the carrier.

10. Place the skin graft over the wound and trim excess skin. The graft is then secured in place using either staples or sutures (4–0 chromic) or tissue glue.

11. Cover the skin graft with bacitracin and a non-adherent dressing. Place a negative therapy wound dressing device over the graft site; use kerlix and an ace bandage to reinforce the dressing. Alternatively, a bolster can be used which involves placing 3–0 silk sutures around the graft and then wrapping mineral oil soaked cotton balls with xeroform and placing it on top of the graft. The dressing is secured in place by tightly tying the bolster down using the silk sutures.

(a) Waiting at least 5 days prior to first dressing change at graft site is recommended.

12. After the bolster is removed, a non-stick dressing with bacitracin antibiotic ointment is placed over the graft and covered with gauze and ace wrap. The dressing is changed daily until the graft is completely healed. Once it is healed, the graft is moisturized daily with moisturizing ointments.

Donor site care: The ace wrap, gauze, and first non-stick dressing is removed 24 hours after surgery. The xeroform is left in place over the donor site and allowed to dessicate. Once the xeroform is dessicated, no further dressings or wound care is needed. The xeroform will peel off as the donor site epithelializes underneath.

Disclaimers

"The views expressed are those of the [author(s)] [presenter(s)] and do not reflect the official views or policy of the Department of Defense or its Components"

Part XII
Amputations

Chapter 46
Above Knee Amputation (AKA)

Shravan Leonard-Murali

Overview

- Make fishmouth incision, starting with posterior incision as distal as possible
- Identify and isolate greater saphenous vein
- Divide muscles down to bone identifying vessels and nerves, and ligating as they are encountered
- Once dissected down to bone circumferentially, clear the femur with periosteal elevator at proposed level of transection
- Transect femur with oscillating saw
- Obtain hemostasis
- Myopexy is option, then bring posterior and anterior flaps together with fascial sutures, then subcutaneous sutures
- Close skin with interrupted nylon sutures

Clinical Pearls

- Thin skin flaps can lead to ischemia and wound breakdown

S. Leonard-Murali (✉)
Department of Surgery, Henry Ford Hospital/Wayne State University, Detroit, MI, USA
e-mail: smurali@hfhs.org

© Springer Nature Switzerland AG 2020
E. Karamanos (ed.), *Common Surgeries Made Easy*,
https://doi.org/10.1007/978-3-030-41350-7_46

277

- Unretracted nerves can become neuromas and lead to chronic pain
- Rough bone edges or protruding bone can lead to pressure sores and wound breakdown
- Be cognizant of intraoperative fluid resuscitation, as edema postoperatively can lead to dehiscence
- 30% of patients become ambulatory postoperatively

Anesthesia

Spinal or epidural anesthesia offers reliable pain control, with an option to leave the catheter in place post-operatively for a few days to aid with recovery. A peripheral nerve block of the sciatic nerve and lumbar plexus/femoral nerve is another good choice, with an option to leave an analgesic pump in place post-operatively. One must consider if the patient is anticoagulated, and, if stronger DVT prophylaxis is desired post-operatively, whether it is safe to leave the analgesic catheters in place.

In diabetics with severe neuropathy, it is sometimes possible to perform an amputation under sedation. This is a viable option, as it can be converted quickly to general anesthesia.

If these options are contraindicated, general anesthesia must be induced.

Positioning

Place the patient supine, with arms to sides, and all bony prominences cushioned. Ensure the table is wide enough to accommodate both limbs with enough room to prep and drape the affected side.

Choice of the skin preparation will depend on the presence or absence of any open wounds. Chlorhexidine/alcohol mixture preparation sticks are appropriate in the absence of open wounds. If any open wounds are present, a betadine or chlorhexidine solution scrub is a better choice. It is important to have an assistant with a pair of sterile gloves to assist with mobilizing the limb during preparation. Start by prepping all visible skin while the limb is laid on the table, down distally as far as the limb goes. Once an adequate area of the distal extremity has been prepped, have the assistant grab a distal area and lift the limb off the table. You may then prepare the posterior aspect and ensure circumferential sterility. Make sure to prepare proximally to the groin. Another assistant in a sterile gown and gloves may then place an elastic cover over the distal extremity, and place a drape underneath. The limb can be laid down onto the drape, and the remainder of draping occurs with either universal, or limb-specific "U" drapes to exclude the proximal patient.

The use of a pneumatic tourniquet for above knee amputation is not universally employed as for more distal amputations. If the planned level of amputation is distal on the femur, then a pneumatic tourniquet application may be feasible. Always apply a soft covering around the leg before applying the tourniquet. One may apply the tourniquet before the preparation. If amputating more proximally, one can apply a sterile tourniquet after preparation and draping.

Landmarks/Incision

The most important consideration for an above knee amputation is the selection of the level of the amputation. The femur is long, and changes in caliber at different areas. One should aim to amputate the femur as distally as possible on the diaphysis, without including the metaphysis. An incision close to where the epicondyles are palpable is not recommended.

The skin incision is usually in a fish-mouth orientation, with the corners of the "mouth" located medially and laterally. The goal of the incision is to create skin and muscle flaps that will allow coverage of the bony end with adequate cushioning and no tension. The anterior and posterior incisions should be very similar, and measurement with a piece of suture is recommended to prevent asymmetry of the flaps.

Operation

1. Begin by turning on the tourniquet after compressing the distal leg with a rubber wrap to aid in the venous return. Test the tourniquet by visualizing pressure changes when you squeeze the leg.
2. Use a 10-blade scalpel to make your fish-mouth incision, with a goal to cut cleanly through the dermis, subcutaneous tissue and fascia. Begin with your posterior incision to keep the anterior field clean. Identify and ligate the greater saphenous vein during dissection (Fig. 46.1).
3. Divide the muscle to bone with cautery, taking care to identify the superficial femoral artery and femoral vein(s), femoral nerve, sciatic nerve or its branches (tibial, peroneal, sural nerves).

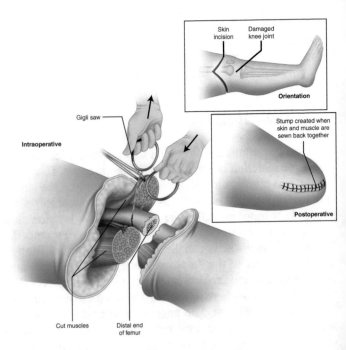

FIGURE 46.1 Incisions for above knee amputation

4. Pull the nerves into field, ligate with an absorbable suture, and transect sharply. Allow nerves to retract and ensure they do not lay in regions where they may scar or be exposed to pressure.

5. Clamp and ligate the arteries and veins mentioned. Silk ties, either free or stick, may be used.

6. Identify the femur and clear the soft tissue circumferentially off the area of the proposed amputation, ensuring this is proximal to the skin incision.

7. Flex the patient's hip to see how the skin relates to the proposed area of amputation. If it retracts too much, choose a more proximal location for the femoral transection.

8. Use a periosteal elevator to further clean the area of the proposed amputation circumferentially.

9. For the femoral transection, an oscillating power saw is most often used. Orient the saw tip perpendicular to the femur surface, with the horizontal axis perpendicular to the femur axis.

10. When using the saw, be sure to brace the base to prevent kicking of the saw. Consistent, firm pressure of the saw against the femur while engaged is required for a clean transection.

11. Have an assistant wet the saw with saline during engagement to keep it cool and limit spread of bone dust.

12. After the femoral transection, an electrocautery device and bone glue may aid in hemostasis from the exposed marrow.

13. Pass the distal end (specimen) off the field.

14. Let down the tourniquet if it is in use, achieve hemostasis with an electrocautery device and ties.

15. Smooth the edges of the cut proximal femur.

16. Myopexy is optional, and may be performed by suturing adductor muscles to the periosteum of the femur to prevent a postoperative abduction/flexion.

17. Reapproximate the fascia with an absorbable suture.

18. Reapproximate the subcutaneous tissues with an absorbable suture if needed.

19. If any tension occurs during the reapproximation of the skin, interrupted full-thickness nylon sutures are recommended.
20. Deep dermal absorbable sutures and staples may be used for the skin if there is no tension.
21. Dress the wound with sterile gauze and a Kerlix wrap. Place wrapped stump in a soft, bulky dressing to prevent post-operative trauma.
22. After a few days a stump-shrinker may be applied to reduce edema.

Chapter 47
Below Knee Amputation (BKA)

Imran Ahmad

Overview

- Make anterior incision as distal as possible, but at least 10 cm distal to tibial tuberosity
- Posterior incision should be made distal to anterior incision for adequate muscle flap coverage of bone
- Divide muscles down to tibia and fibula identifying anterior tibial vessels and nerves, and ligating them as they are encountered
- Once dissected down to bone circumferentially, clear the tibia and fibula with periosteal elevator at proposed level of transection
- Transect bones with oscillating saw
- Obtain hemostasis
- Suture superficial posterior compartment to periosteum of tibia for muscle flap coverage, then place deep dermal sutures
- Close skin with nylon horizontal sutures

I. Ahmad (✉)
Department of General Surgery, Henry Ford Hospital/Wayne State University, Detroit, MI, USA
e-mail: iahmad1@hfhs.org

© Springer Nature Switzerland AG 2020
E. Karamanos (ed.), *Common Surgeries Made Easy*,
https://doi.org/10.1007/978-3-030-41350-7_47

Clinical Pearls

- Thin skin flaps can lead to ischemia and wound breakdown
- Unretracted nerves can lead to chronic pain
- Rough bone edges or protruding bone can lead to pressure soars and wound breakdown
- Be cognizant of intraoperative fluid resuscitation, as edema postoperatively can lead to dehiscence
- 70% of patients become ambulatory postoperatively
- Begin physical therapy as soon as possible to avoid knee contractures

Patient Position

The patient is placed supine with arms secured and the lower extremities at the end of the bed. A foley catheter is not required. Prep the limb circumferentially with a chloraprep. Prep should include the proximal thigh to the distal foot. A "wet prep" of either betadine or chlorhexidine (Hibiclens) may be used in areas of infection or open wounds. Drape in a sterile fashion. If there is an isolated area of infection, an impervious barrier should be used to exclude the area prior to draping. Place several layers of web roll circumferentially around the proximal thigh followed by a sterile tourniquet. The limb may be exsanguinated using elastic compression such as an Esmarch. However, the use of an Esmarch is not recommended in settings of infections. Furthermore, tourniquets are not recommended in settings of ischemic disease. If tourniquet is indicated, it is insufflated to 1.5–2.0× the patient's systolic pressure.

Anesthesia

Spinal anesthesia versus a peripheral nerve block may be used with monitored anesthesia care (MAC) during the procedure. If unavailable, general anesthesia should be performed.

Operative Steps

1. The purpose of the skin incision is to mark the level of amputation and create a long posterior flap. The skin should be marked 10 cm distal to the tibial tuberosity (Fig. 47.1).

2. Perform the skin incision 2 cm distal to planned tibial transection site. The anterior skin incision should encompass 2/3 of the total leg circumference. From the edges of the anterior incision, the posterior flap should be created distally. The length of the posterior flap should be 1/3 of the total leg circumference. The skin incision should include the skin and the fascia and the posterior flap

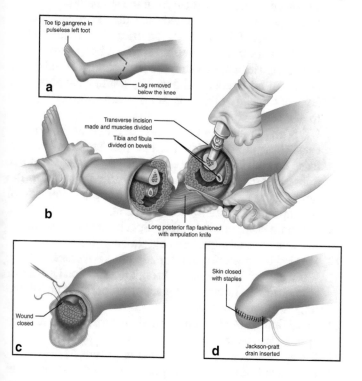

FIGURE 47.1 Below knee amputation

should be slightly curved. Care should be taken to identify and ligate the great saphenous vein during the medial incision.

3. Divide the anterior and lateral compartment down to the tibia and fibula. Take care to dissect the anterior tibial neurovascular bundle. Tie the anterior tibial artery proximally, distally, and divide the artery. Further suture ligation of the anterior tibial artery may be performed. Sharply divide the deep peroneal nerve as proximal as possible for adequate retraction.

4. Lift the anterior skin edge using rake retractors to expose the tibia at the level of planned transection. A periosteal elevator should be used to circumferentially separate the periosteum to at least 2 cm from the skin edge.

5. Use a powered saw to divide the tibia perpendicular to the long axis of the bone. The anterior tibia should be beveled till smooth via a powered saw or a bone rasp.

6. Using a periosteal elevator, the periosteum should be circumferentially separated from the fibula 2 cm above the level of the end of the tibia. A bone cutter should be used to divide the fibula.

7. Using an amputation knife transect the posterior soft tissues. The knife should be used perpendicular to the limb axis to divide the deep posterior compartment. Subsequently, the knife should be turned parallel to the limb axis to create a posterior flap using the contents of the superficial posterior compartment.

8. The limb is amputated and the specimen is handed off.

9. Release the tourniquet and obtain hemostasis.

10. Fashion the posterior flap for adequate coverage.

11. With an absorbable suture, bring the superficial posterior compartment fascia to the anterior periosteum of the tibia for bone coverage.

12. Place interrupted deep dermal absorbable sutures to approximate skin edges.

13. Close the skin with staples or nylon sutures.

14. Place a soft and bulky compression dressing around the stump. The use of a knee immobilizer is discouraged at this step because of concerns for pressure injuries.

Anatomy

Anterior Compartment
- *m:* Tibialis anterior, extensor muscles of the foot, and fibularis (peroneus) tertius muscles.
- *a:* Anterior tibial artery.
- *n:* Deep fibular (peroneal) nerve.

Lateral Compartment
- *m:* Fibularis (peroneus) longus and fibularis (peroneus) brevis muscles.
- *a:* Superficial fibular (peroneal) nerve.

Superficial Posterior Compartment
- *m:* Gastrocnemius, soleus, and plantaris muscles.
- *a:* The arteries which supply these muscles descend from the popliteal artery. The sural arteries.
- *n:* Tibial nerve branches supply these muscles.

Deep Posterior Compartment
- *m:* Tibialis posterior, flexor muscles of the foot and popliteus muscles.
- *a:* Posterior tibial and fibular (peroneal) arteries.
- *n:* Tibial nerve.

Chapter 48
Toe/Ray Amputation

Shravan Leonard-Murali

Overview

- Make a racquet incision and deepen it to bone; ensure handle aspect is dorsal, not lateral
- Incise tendon off bone, and determine level of amputation, and use ronguer or bone cutter to amputate. If level of amputation at the joint, use a 15 blade scalpel to cut into the joint capsule
- Grasp distal bone and dislocate
- If performing ray amputation, dissect metatarsal and transect through shaft
- Smooth proximal edge of metatarsal
- Ensure hemostasis and close skin

Clinical Pearls

- Ankle blocks are quick, easy, and effective
- Make a conservative incision first, you can always trim excess skin at conclusion of case

S. Leonard-Murali (✉)
Department of Surgery, Henry Ford Hospital/Wayne State University, Detroit, MI, USA
e-mail: smurali@hfhs.org

© Springer Nature Switzerland AG 2020
E. Karamanos (ed.), *Common Surgeries Made Easy*,
https://doi.org/10.1007/978-3-030-41350-7_48

289

- Avoid lateral toes as vessels/nerves run here
- 1st toe amputation has the greatest impact, the 3rd toe has the least impact
- Deciding between toe and ray amputation depends on whether distal tissue is viable or not

Anesthesia

General anesthesia is rarely needed for isolated toe/ray amputations. An ankle block is effective and spares patients from the use of sedatives and narcotics. This involves a local anesthetic injection of two deep nerves (deep peroneal, posterior tibial), and three superficial nerves (superficial peroneal, sural, saphenous). If the distal phalanx is the only bone being amputated, a toe block may be sufficient, but a full ankle block is recommended.

Positioning

Patients can be placed supine, or with the head of the bed up to 30–40° since they often do not require sedatives or narcotics with ankle blocks. Ensure there is enough working area to isolate the foot in question, and place a pneumatic tourniquet on the ipsilateral thigh. Although tourniquets on the leg may be partially effective, they often cannot achieve enough compression between the tibia and fibula to completely halt the blood flow. Always apply a soft covering between the skin and the tourniquet.

If the skin is intact, a simple chlorhexidine/alcohol based preparation may be sufficient. Otherwise, a wet preparation with iodine or chlorhexidine solution is recommended to sterilize the entire foot and leg up to the mid-calf. In either case, an assistant will be necessary. They will wear sterile gloves and grasp the foot at a prepped area, raise the leg in the air, allow the preparation to be completed circumferentially, and then allow a sterile drape to be placed underneath. An extremity drape is useful to wrap tightly around the calf. Blue towels may also be used to wrap around the calf circumferentially and maintain the sterile field.

Landmarks/Incision

The preservation of enough skin for coverage of the stumps is the single most technically important aspect of the procedure. A "racquet" incision is most often used for toe and ray amputations, with the "head" being a circumferential incision distal to the level of the intended bone amputation level, and the "handle" being a longitudinal incision on the dorsal aspect extending proximally. For ray amputations the "handle" is extended onto the metatarsal shaft. A "U" shaped incision is made on the plantar aspect, ensuring all ulcers and ischemic skin are included.

Operation

1. Begin by compressing the foot with rubber wrap to aid in venous return.
2. Follow this with activation of the tourniquet. Test the tourniquet by visualizing pressure changes when you squeeze the foot/leg.
3. Use a 15-blade or a 10-blade scalpel to make a "racquet" incision. Make the incision down to the bone, incising any tendon in the way. Ensure that your "handle" incision is dorsal, and not lateral, as the vessels/nerves will lie lateral.
4. After the skin and soft tissue are incised and the tendons have been cut and allowed to retract, find the level of the bone you would like to amputate.
5. Use a bone cutter and/or rongeurs to cut and trim the bone appropriately.
6. Smooth the edges of the bone after cutting to reduce the risk of pressure ulceration to the intended skin coverage.
7. If an amputation at the level of the joint is desired, use a 15-blade scalpel to cut into the joint capsule and cut any fibrous attachments between the bones.
8. Firmly grasp the distal bone and dislocate. If the original incision was successful, the specimen should be free to be passed off the field.

9. Use rongeurs to clean off the proximal bone, removing any residual cartilage.
10. For a ray amputation, simply extend the "handle" incision proximally, transect the metatarsal through shaft, and smooth the proximal metatarsal end.
11. Ensure hemostasis with electrocautery, balancing hemostasis with the risk of inducing ischemia. Turn off the tourniquet before closure to reevaluate.
12. Close the skin with full-thickness non-absorbable, monofilament interrupted sutures, or leave open if done for infection.
13. Dress with gauze and Kerlix wrap. If left open, apply damp gauze to the wound, then wrap with a Kerlix. There is no advantage to using iodine soaked gauze versus saline.

Part XIII
Miscellaneous

Chapter 49
Percutaneous Dilatational Tracheostomy

Semeret T. Munie and Arielle Hodari Gupta

Overview

- Introduce bronchoscope through ET tube
- Assess trachea, bronchi, and carina
- Deflate ET tube balloon, and withdraw ET tube proximal to 2nd or 3rd tracheal ring
- Make skin incision over site of tracheostomy
- Using large bore needle, introduce under direct visualization into trachea
- Use seldinger technique to advance wire, and then serially dilate the skin and soft tissue tract
- Advance the tracheostomy over the dilator into the trachea under direct visualization
- Remove dilator, and put inner cannula in tracheostomy, and connect to vent
- Ensure adequate tidal volumes, no air leak, and then remove ET tube

S. T. Munie
Division of Bariatric and Minimally Invasive Surgery, Medical College of Wisconsin, Milwaukee, WI, USA

A. H. Gupta (✉)
Department of Surgery, Henry Ford Hospital/Wayne State University, Detroit, MI, USA
e-mail: agupta12@hfhs.org

© Springer Nature Switzerland AG 2020
E. Karamanos (ed.), *Common Surgeries Made Easy*,
https://doi.org/10.1007/978-3-030-41350-7_49

Clinical Pearls

- Tracheostomy placed too high will result in tracheal stenosis
- Tracheostomy placed too low results in increased risk of tracheoinominate fistula
- Tracheoinominate fistula

  - Will have sentinel bleed prior to life threatening bleed
  - CTA can be diagnostic, but may miss fistula
  - Bronchoscopy may be difficult to visualize due to blood in trachea; need to intubate from above, and withdraw the tube and scopeto assess the ET tube insertion site

- Able to wean patients off vent quicker because they need less sedation

Patient Positioning

Supine, arms adducted.

A shoulder roll should be placed between the shoulder blades hyperextending the neck unless there is concern for a cervical spine injury.

A bronchoscopy tower to be set up opposite of the proceduralist.

Chlorahexidine prep. No foley needed.

Team Members

The bronchoscopist at the head of bed.

Proceduralist: if right handed, he/she will stand at the right of the patient. If left handed, he/she should stand to the left of the patient.

Anesthesia

Pulse oximetry, blood pressure monitoring and telemetry monitoring are mandatory.

Place the patient on 100% oxygenation on a full vent support setting.

Medications being administered will include analgesics and a sedative to induce deep sedation to be followed by a paralytic medication.

Operative Steps

1. Palpate the neck to identify important landmarks: thyroid cartilage notch, cricoid cartilage and sternal notch. The access point for the tracheostomy should be between the first and second or the second and third tracheal cartilage.
2. After local anesthetics with 1% Lidocaine at the desired anatomic location, make a 1.5–2 cm transverse incision with care taken to not injure the vessels underneath the skin.
3. Insert the bronchoscope through the ET tube and position approximately 1–2 cm proximal to the tip of the tube.
4. Deflate the balloon of the ET tube and withdraw to the desired location above the insertion site while still in the trachea.
5. If the ET tube accidentally gets dislodged from the vocal cords, DO NOT PANIC!! Just advance the bronchoscope forward through the cords and slide the ET tube over it to secure the airway.
6. Use the introducer needle located in the kit to enter the trachea at the 12 o'clock location while observing with the bronchoscope. BE CAREFUL NOT TO PUNCTURE THE BACK WALL OF THE TRACHEA.

7. Advance the J tip wire through the needle under direct visualization to ensure the back wall is not injured.
8. Remove the needle. Use the introducer dilator to dilate the tract over the wire.
9. Place the white guide catheter along with the Blue Rhino advanced dilator until the thick black line is observed on the endoscope. Use one handed technique.
10. Remove the Blue Rhino dilator, but leave the white guide catheter on the wire.
11. Place the tracheostomy tube along with the appropriate size loading dilator over the wire into the trachea. The loading dilator, guide catheter and wire are all removed together while the tracheostomy is held in position.
12. The inner cannula is placed and the ventilator circuit is moved from the ET tube to the Trach.
13. Observe quickly for return of expiratory tidal volume on the ventilator machine as well as confirm correct positioning by performing a bronchoscopy through the tracheostomy.
14. The tracheostomy is secured in place with sutures and a neck collar.
15. A routine chest x-ray to confirm tracheostomy position after procedure is not necessary unless there were issues during the procedure.

Chapter 50
Percutaneous Endoscopic Gastrostomy (PEG) Tube Placement

Semeret T. Munie and Arielle Hodari Gupta

Overview

- Advance gastroscope into esophagus, and then into stomach
- Insufflate stomach until rugae flatten out
- Advance scope to greater curvature of stomach and perform transillumination
- Assistant will then palpate on abdominal wall at site of transillumination
- 1:1 differentiation with palpation
- Make 1 cm skin incision over chosen site, and advance large bore needle under direct visualization
- Assistant should hold negative pressure and see bubbles in syringe at same time endoscopist sees needle in stomach

S. T. Munie
Division of Bariatric and Minimally Invasive Surgery, Medical College of Wisconsin, Milwaukee, WI, USA

A. H. Gupta (✉)
Department of Surgery, Henry Ford Hospital/Wayne State University, Detroit, MI, USA
e-mail: agupta12@hfhs.org

© Springer Nature Switzerland AG 2020
E. Karamanos (ed.), *Common Surgeries Made Easy*,
https://doi.org/10.1007/978-3-030-41350-7_50

299

- Advance wire in seldinger technique, and snagged by endoscopist, and scope and wire withdrawn
- Attach PEG to wire and assistant pulls PEG into stomach
- Gastroscope re-advanced into stomach to assess that PEG is not too tight on stomach wall

Clinical Pearls

- Do not sinch PEG down too tight, as this will lead to buried bumper syndrome
- If having trouble with transillumination, or appropriate differentiation with palpation, proceed to laparoscopic or open gastrostomy tube placement
- If PEG dislodged within 72 hours, patient requires surgical intervention with open gastrostomy tube

  - If after 72 hours may be amenable to repeat endoscopy and tube placement

- If PEG dislodged more than a few weeks after placement, replace bedside, and shoot contrast study

Patient Positioning

The procedure can be safely performed at the bedside in the ICU or in the operating room. The patient should be placed in the supine position with the arms at the patient's side.

All clothes and objects should be removed from the patient's abdomen.

An EGD tower and a scope with proper function should be checked before the start of the endoscopy.

Position the EGD tower at the right side of the patient.

A bite block is needed.

Personal protective equipment should be used by the endoscopist and a sterile gown, mask and head covers should be used by the person performing the abdominal portion of the procedure.

Chlorhexidine prep. No foley needed.

Team Members

Three individuals are needed for procedure:

- An endoscopist at the head of the bed.
- An endoscopist assistant at the head of bed to control snare.
- Proceduralist on the left side of the patient.

An additional individual performing the sedation and monitoring the vital signs might be needed based on individual practices for sedation.

Anesthesia

The patient should be NPO with any tube feeds held prior to the procedure. If an NG tube is already in place, connect it to suction prior to the start of the procedure.

If the patient is having both a tracheostomy and a PEG performed at the same time, it is preferable to perform the tracheostomy first to avoid an accidental dislodgement of the endotracheal tube with manipulation of the mouth for the endoscopy.

Continuous pulse oximetry, blood pressure monitoring as well as telemetry monitoring are recommended.

Bedside procedural sedation can be given with a combination of analgesic and sedative medications. If the procedure is being performed in a non-intubated patient, the use of a trained anesthesiologist dedicated to monitoring patient's airway is recommended.

Operative Steps

1. The endoscopist at the head of the bed begins the EGD by placing the endoscope through the bite block into the mouth and advances the scope through the esophagus into the stomach.
2. Insufflate the stomach fully until the folds in the mucosa flatten out, allowing the stomach to lay flush against the abdominal wall.
3. The proceduralist on the left of the patient pushes the left upper quadrant of the abdomen two finger width inferior to the costal margin, while at the same time looking at the endoscopy screen to see the corresponding invagination of the stomach
4. Two checks should be performed to ensure there is no bowel between the stomach and abdominal wall. One-to-one touch differentiation as well as transillumination HAVE TO BE ACHIEVED. IF THESE TWO SAFETY STEPS ARE NOT MET, PEG PLACEMENT MUST BE ABORTED!!!
5. Chloraprep abdomen and open a PEG kit, put on a sterile gown and gloves. Place the sterile drape included in the kit.
6. Pass off the snare and PEG tube to the endoscopist at the head of the bed.
7. The endoscopist passes the snare through the working port of the EGD until it is observed coming out of the tip of the endoscope screen. The endoscopist's assistant will be ready with the snare to open and close the snare as needed.
8. Locally anesthetize the selected abdominal wall skin with 1% Lidocaine.

9. Make a small 5 mm incision. Insert the PEG needle through the abdominal wall into the stomach while directly visualizing through the endoscopy. Pass the PEG wire through the needle into the stomach and grab it with the snare.

10. Pull the wire and the endoscope out through the mouth while keeping hold of the wire at the abdominal wall.

11. The end of the PEG tube is looped through the wire and secured.

12. Using the pull technique, the wire is pulled back out through the abdominal wall along with the PEG tube.

13. The correct position of the PEG is confirmed by endoscopy.

14. The bumper, clamp and PEG tip are connected to the PEG tube, making sure not to make the bumper too tight, which will result in tissue necrosis.

Chapter 51
Abdominal Access for Laparoscopic Surgery

Heath J. Antoine

Preoperative Evaluation

Prior to any operation, review the patient's medical and surgical history. Determine if there are any contraindications to laparoscopic surgery such as inability to tolerate pneumoperitoneum due to impaired cardiovascular reserve or hemodynamic instability, acute intestinal obstruction with very dilated bowels, or uncorrected coagulopathies.

Ascertain what prior surgeries the patient has undergone to anticipate where probable adhesions may exist.

Physically examine the abdomen for scars or hernias and review relevant imaging.

Have the patient urinate in the preoperative holding area prior to surgery to decompress the bladder, unless a Foley catheter will be placed intra-operatively.

H. J. Antoine (✉)
Robert Wood Johnson University Hospital,
New Brunswick, NJ, USA

© Springer Nature Switzerland AG 2020
E. Karamanos (ed.), *Common Surgeries Made Easy*,
https://doi.org/10.1007/978-3-030-41350-7_51

Intraoperative Preparation

Have the anesthesiologist place an orogastric or nasogastric tube following intubation to empty gastric contents and reduce stomach distension.

Ensure that the camera and light source are working and that the carbon dioxide tanks are full.

The access point should be chosen in a location felt to be the safest, farthest from adhesions, and useful for your particular laparoscopic procedure. Knowledge of abdominal wall anatomy and familiarity with both open and closed entry techniques are essential.

Anatomy of the Abdominal Wall

- *Abdominal Wall Vessels*: The superior epigastric artery and vein traverses the abdomen bilaterally from rostral to caudal several cm off of midline in the rectus sheath and anastomose with the inferior epigastric artery and vein. Additional flow to the abdominal wall from superficial and deep iliac circumflex arteries is found in the hypogastrium.
- *Umbilicus*: The umbilicus is a midline fascial structure that loses its primary function after birth. At the umbilicus, the median umbilical ligament (obliterated urachus) and medial umbilical ligaments (obliterated umbilical arteries) come together to form the thickened fascia. An umbilical hernia is a defect in this fascia and entry here is discouraged.
- *Layers of the Abdominal Wall*: The outermost layer of the abdominal wall is the skin, which is followed by subcutaneous tissue (Camper's superficial fatty layer and Scarpa's deep membranous layers of fascia), followed by several myofascial layers (different above and below the arcuate line), preperitoneal fat, and lastly peritoneum.

"Closed" Veress Needle Technique for Insufflation

The use of the Veress needle is the oldest known technique for insufflation with carbon dioxide in laparoscopy. It is designed to hold a dull spring-loaded stylet that is pushed back as it enters the skin and fascial layers to expose a beveled cutting needle. When the tip of the needle enters the peritoneal cavity, the dull stylet springs forward protecting the abdominal contents below. The most common access site for insufflation with a Veress needle is at the umbilicus since there is no fat or muscle between the skin and the peritoneum; however, entry at Palmer's point (see below) is a much safer location. Entry at the umbilicus is contraindicated when the patient has an umbilical hernia or suspicion of underlying adhesions.

1. Infiltrate the skin with a local anesthetic agent.
2. A small skin incision is made either infra or supra-umbilically to accommodate either the Veress needle or a port of desired size.
3. Verify that the Veress is working properly and that there is appropriate retraction of the tip.
4. Grasp the fascia or umbilical stalk with forceps or a Kocher clamp if you are able, and insert the Veress through the linea alba. Hold the Veress like a dart by the shaft for the best control. Do not try to elevate the skin alone, as it has been associated with increased complications.
5. As the needle moves through the layers of the abdominal wall, the surgeon will hear and feel a click as the protective sheath recoils back in place when it has crossed a fascial layer and the peritoneum. Generally, the surgeon will hear and feel 2 clicks, one for the abdominal fascia and one for the peritoneum at this location.
6. To confirm entry, attach a syringe filled with saline (with plunger removed) directly to the Veress needle. Entry is confirmed if the saline flows freely through the needle into the peritoneal cavity.

7. One can also aspirate to look for blood, bowel contents, or urine.
8. However, many surgeons will simply attach the insufflation tubing at a low flow level and look for an opening pressure less than 8–10 mmHg. If it is greater than 10 mmHg in a non-obese patient, gently withdraw the catheter as it can become adherent to the underlying omentum or adhesions. If you have withdrawn it entirely (will often see bubbling at the incision site indicating you are above the fascia), then attempt to insert the needle again after confirming adequate gas flow through it. If you are not successful after two attempts, move to another location or try using an open Hasson technique (see below).

Although the most common site of insertion of the Veress needle is at the umbilicus, Raoul Palmer, who pioneered its use in 1947, advocated for its insertion 3 cm below the left subcostal border at the midclavicular line (Palmer's point). He reasoned that in thin individuals, the aorta and IVC lie below the umbilicus and in obese patients, the umbilicus is shifted caudally to the level of the aortic bifurcation. It is very common in foregut and bariatric surgery to use Palmer's point to insufflate with the Veress needle. At Palmer's point, 4 clicks will be appreciated as you traverse the now separated fascial layers and peritoneum. In practice, grasping of the underlying fascia prior to insertion of the Veress needle is not required at this location as there is no underlying bowel, the left lobe of the liver is smaller than the right, and the spleen is located more posteriorly.

1. To place the port once fully insufflated (15 mmHg, or 2–5 L of CO_2), remove the Veress needle and insert the port along this track.
2. Use a gentle twisting motion (180-degree rotations) to advance the trocar, with care taken to keep your index finger extended to stop forward momentum should the fascia suddenly give way.
3. Likewise, the port can be placed away from the Veress entry at another location.

4. Once the port is inserted, opening the valve should elicit a rush of gas.
5. Remove the insert and place the laparoscope through the cannula and inspect for possible underlying damage.
6. The remainder of the ports will now be placed under direct visualization.

"Closed" Optical Trocar Entry

Rather than placement of a trocar blindly after insufflation, the use of an optical trocar in conjunction with a 0-degree laparoscope will allow for direct entry of the abdomen with visualization. As above, most commonly a Veress needle is used to create pneumoperitoneum. Some surgeons will use an optical trocar for entry without prior insufflation, however this is not advised.

1. Advance the laparoscope into the port and adjust the focus to the tip of the trocar.
2. Apply a continuous, gentle twisting pressure with finger extended to advance the scope.
3. Visually, the subcutaneous fat will be noted first followed by at least two muscle layers and lastly the peritoneum depending on where the site of entry is.
4. Once through the fascia, direct the tip towards an open portion of the abdomen as it goes through the peritoneum to avoid injuring any intra-abdominal organs or blood vessels.
5. Once through the peritoneum, you will see either black (air) or intra-abdominal contents.
6. The safest location for entry using an optical trocar is at Palmer's point in the left upper quadrant. However, it can also be used just off midline to be able to visualize the abdominal musculature, or even in the right upper quadrant with care taken not to injure the underlying liver or gallbladder.

"Open" Hasson Technique

When concerned about injury to bowel due to adhesions from prior operations, many will advocate for using an open technique for trocar insertion.

1. In the open Hasson technique, a small skin incision is made at the umbilicus following infiltration with local.
2. Next, using two S retractors, the subcutaneous tissue is pushed aside to dissect down to the rectus fascia. Some will use a Kelly to spread the subcutaneous tissue prior to retracting it.
3. The fascia is grasped with a Kocher clamp and elevated.
4. Stay sutures (0 Vicryl or similar absorbable suture) are placed through the fascia.
5. The fascia is then opened with a scalpel to expose the pre-peritoneal fat.
6. The underlying peritoneum is elevated using two tonsil clamps and a scalpel is used again to make a small nick in the peritoneum.
7. Next, a smaller S retractor is inserted into this space to confirm entry into the peritoneum. A finger can be used to feel the undersurface of the peritoneum to confirm the anatomy and to clear away neighboring adhesions.
8. A trocar is then inserted directly into this space.
9. A Hasson port is designed to allow for the fascial sutures to be secured directly to the port. If the Hasson port has a balloon tip, inflate it to prevent accidental port dislodgement.
10. Connect the carbon dioxide and insufflate the abdomen to 15 mm Hg.
11. At the end of the case, the stay sutures can be used to aid in placement of better fascial sutures or to close the fascial defect directly.

Troubleshooting

- If the Veress is placed and there is no free flow of saline or a high opening pressure when connected to carbon dioxide, initially try to withdraw the Veress needle slowly in case the tip is abutting bowel, omentum, or not in the peritoneal cavity.
- If the pressure remains high, remove the Veress needle and attempt a second pass.
- If you are not comfortable with the insufflation pressures or the results of the saline drop test, do not continue with insufflation. Complication rates following unsuccessful insertion attempts rise dramatically on the second and third try.
- If you are unsuccessful with a Veress needle approach, move to another location or attempt a different method of entry.

Chapter 52
Facial Lacerations

Adam Wandell

Introduction

Soft tissue injuries to the face actually do not require immediate closure because of immense vascular supply of the face. Clean wounds may be closed primarily up to 2 days following after initial injury; however, it is ideal to close any facial laceration within 24 hours of initial injury. During the initial exam and assessment, the tissue should be kept moist with gauze soaked preferably in antibiotic solution. During initial examination it is also important to document if any vital structures have been damaged, including any nerves, major vessels, or ducts.

Tetanus

For unimmunized patients = give passive immunization with hyperimmune tetanus globulin + active tetanus immunization.

A. Wandell (✉)
Department of Oral and Maxillofacial Surgery, UT Health San Antonio, San Antonio, TX, USA
e-mail: Wandell@uthscsa.edu

© Springer Nature Switzerland AG 2020
E. Karamanos (ed.), *Common Surgeries Made Easy*,
https://doi.org/10.1007/978-3-030-41350-7_52

For previous immunized patients, but not within 10 years = give a booster dose of 0.5 mL of tetanus toxoid.

Steps

1. Thoroughly examine and inspect the wound for any possible foreign bodies.
2. Anesthetize the area with lidocaine 1% with epinephrine 1:100 k (except on or near nose near, do not use epinephrine); max dose = 7 mg/kg

   - Use 25 gauge needle or smaller.
   - Insert needle into the wound margin subcutaneous tissue (as opposed to penetrating skin).

3. Debride any nonviable tissue, remove any foreign fragments, and create a clean bed for closure.
4. Obtain Hemostasis with firm pressure with a sterile gauze.
5. Use copious irrigation (3 L) of normal saline irrigation.
6. Approximate muscles and deep layers first; use 3–0; 4–0 resorbable sutures (recommend = Vicryl non-dyed braided) for deep layers.
7. Approximate skin without tension, relaxed margins, eliminate dead space; use (5–0, 6,0) sutures (recommend Prolene if patient likely to return to clinic or Fast Gut suture if patient follow up is questionable)

   - The skin sutures should be placed 2 mm from wound margin.
   - The goal is to create proper tissue eversion to minimize scar while collagen fibers contract during wound healing.

8. Consider various topical medications and ointments (recommend opthalmic bacitracin).
9. Remove any non-resorbable sutures at 5–7 days follow up.
10. Dermabrasion may be performed at 4–8 week mark; or a scar revision at 6 months.

Pearls and Pitfalls

The two most common reasons for suture scars are closing the wound under tension and delayed removal of the sutures.

The width of the scar is proportional to the amount of tension needed in order to close the wound.

Usually, the scar is given time to mature (6–12 months) before any revision surgery is considered.

Index

© Springer Nature Switzerland AG 2020
E. Karamanos (ed.), *Common Surgeries Made Easy*,
https://doi.org/10.1007/978-3-030-41350-7